THE LAST CHILDHOOD

CARRIE KNOWLES

RTP

Research Triangle Publishing, Inc.

Published by
Research Triangle Publishing, Inc.
PO Box 1130
Fuquay-Varina, NC 27526

ISBN 1-884570-67-4

Cover Design by Kathy Holbrook

Library of Congress Catalog Card Number: 97-65321

Printed in the United States of America
10 9 8 7 6 5 4 3 2 1

For my grandmother,

Laura Isabelle Barr

my mother,

Ruth Margaret Powers

and my sister,

Laura Ruth Mindel,
who carries the names
of her mother and grandmother
with dignity and spirit.

I feel lucky she is my sister.

ACKNOWLEDGMENTS

I would like to thank Sy Safransky for publishing the original piece, "The Only Child" (now chapter 3), in his fine publication, *The Sun*, August 1993. His comments and enthusiasm gave me the confidence I needed to write more.

Shortly after "The Only Child" was published, the North Carolina Arts Council generously awarded me a Literary Nonfiction Writer's Project Grant to complete work on this book. The North Carolina Arts Council is a state agency. Its funds for grants come from both the National Endowment for the Arts and the North Carolina State Legislature. Debbie McGill, director of the NCAC Literature Section, through the financial thick and thin of funding, has managed to support and encourage more writers than should be humanly possible. Thank you.

A special thanks to my brothers, Gary and Charles, and my sister, Lolly, who asked me to write this book and lovingly and generously gave me permission to tell our story.

Although I do not know them all, thanks to everyone who works at the Chelsea Methodist Home and other special facilities across the country providing safe, caring places for people like my mother.

Also, many thanks to Dr. Marjorie Carr who took time from her busy medical practice to read this book and give suggestions and support. And, to my good friend Peggy Payne, who unfailingly eats lunch with me every week at Ballantine's and who manages to see me through rough drafts and rough times with sound guidance and good humor.

Thanks also to Bonnie Tilson and Elizabeth and David Anderson, the three best people I know to work with if you feel compelled to publish a book. And Georgann Eubanks who is ever so good at convincing you you've done the right thing.

And last, but hardly least, many thanks to my best friend/copy editor/husband Jeff Leiter, who had no idea what he was getting into when he married a writer but stayed with me anyway. And to our three children: Neil Barr, Hedy Ellis, and Samuel "Cole" Leiter, who are my toughest critics when it comes to dinner, but my most enthusiastic supporters when it comes to my work.

Thank you all.

PROLOGUE

LAST NIGHT I DREAMED MY MOTHER KNEW MY NAME. IT was one of those dreams where you feel yourself struggling to scramble up from the well of sleep into the real world so you can use the knowledge you've just gained. When morning mercifully came, I wanted more than anything to get up, get dressed, go to the airport, fly to Michigan, and see if it were true.

If it were, I didn't know quite what I'd do. In my dream, I sat and talked to my mother. I pushed her in her wheelchair around the hospital and we looked out the windows. She introduced me to her friends. We had a fine visit. She showed me her right leg and told me where it hurt. She explained to me, like we had explained to her, that she couldn't walk anymore because her brain and foot no longer talked to each other. I helped her into bed and propped her leg up on a pillow so she would be comfortable. I looked for the doctor and asked if there were pain medicines he could give her. I called my sister and told her Mom knew my name and was our mother again.

In my dream, my sister came and saw for herself. She was as relieved as I was to discover Mom was, except for her leg, fine. Mom said she liked the hospital where she lived. She said the people were good to her and her room was comfortable.

I remember crying once in the dream when I told my mother I was sorry I had quit writing her. I confessed I had not written since I had last seen her because I had found all my cards and letters unopened in the drawer of her nightstand. That was the true part of the dream: I had found my letters and cards unopened in her room, and since then had been unable to force myself to write her. I had not made a conscious decision to quit, but realized as Valentine's Day rolled by, I had forgotten to send her a card. A week later, when I found the card I had bought for her but failed to send, I sat in my office and cried.

I was able to dismiss the part of the dream about not writing my mother, because it happened and I knew how it got in the dream. But, I was shaken by the dream notion that we had failed to notice she was normal again. What gnawed at me all night long was the idea we had quit believing she would get better, so we had quit looking for her to get better. And, maybe, just maybe, we were wrong and she had gotten better and we hadn't noticed.

It was one of those buried-alive dreams: a final exam nightmare where you have forgotten to take the class or can't find the door to get into the room. It was a failure dream. Deep in my dreams I believed I had failed my mother. As irrational as this sense of failure is, I know I am not the only one who feels this way. There are thousands of daughters, sons, and spouses who go to bed each night dreading the dark and its daunting dreams of failure. I also know they go to sleep wondering what horrors the next day of

Alzheimer's will bring them, because Alzheimer's is full of surprises, trials, and tribulations.

Left with no short-term or long-term memory, victims in the later stages of Alzheimer's cannot and do not talk about their disease. We do not know what they are experiencing. The "other victims" of Alzheimer's, however, despite their good intentions and caretaking, wrestle day and night with failure. The failure of overlooking the warning signs of the early stages. Failure to act quickly enough. The failure of not being able to care enough to make a difference, or to stop the disease. The failure to remain memorable enough to be a face and a name their parent or loved one can recall. The failure to be a memory.

But, in order to continue to care and love, you have to believe you haven't failed. You have to accept that you do not have the power to stop the wild progression of the disease and the destruction it leaves in its wake.

When I talked to my sister last week, she told me Mom was moved to a semiprivate room. We had asked for the move because we thought it might help Mom to have someone in the room with her: she had never, until she moved to the Chelsea Methodist Home, slept in a room by herself.

We were relieved a semiprivate room had at last become available and hoped it would help her. Ironically, Mom did not even notice her room had been changed or that someone else was living in it with her.

I was sorry we had pushed for the move. It was unsettling and sobering to discover Mom was so out of touch with reality and her surroundings that she failed to notice she not only had a new room, but someone else living there with her.

I read an article a couple of years ago about an acting agency in Japan offering an unusual service to busy fast-track clients: they provide actors to pose as these clients and visit their parents. Besides money for the service, the clients provide the agency with a profile and picture of themselves and a list of questions the actors should ask their parents to aid in making small talk during the visit. The article made a big deal about the acting agency trying to make good "physical" matches between client and actor to maintain as much of a personal fantasy as possible for the parents.

How do these parents feel knowing they are talking to an actor instead of their real son or daughter? What do the actors think about performing someone else's family obligations for pay? The article didn't elaborate on these issues. Instead, it went on to say, for the Japanese parent, there is the reality of the fantasy. They know they are talking to an actor. They know they are not talking to their child. They know the actor is a fake, and if they want to talk to their real child, all they have to do is call them on the phone.

Where is that phone? Where is that missing piece of technology, that medical magic waiting to hook me up to my mother again? Where is my mother? Where are her children?

There is no fantasy here, no actor playing my mom, just an unsettling truth that the real her no longer exists. I can go visit the woman who looks like my mother, but my visit isn't any more memorable for her than a visit by an actor posing as me. I can hug her and kiss her and talk to her, but she cannot remember me and will not remember I have been there and touched her.

Why does Alzheimer's happen? Why can't we stop it? Will it happen to me?

These dreams and other real-life struggles are why I wrote this book. I hope it helps you think about what may be happening to you or someone you love. I hope my family's experiences help you make some sense out of what you are struggling with as your loved one slips farther and farther away from you. And, I sincerely hope it helps to know you are not alone in this nightmare. More importantly, I hope this book makes you realize you have not failed. You have done your best. The best anyone can do under these strange and powerfully disturbing circumstances.

Chapter One

1991-The year we knew for sure.

THERE IS NOTHING UNUSUAL ABOUT US. WE ARE FOUR siblings: two girls, two boys, all born roughly four or five years apart. My older brother, Gary, born 1945, was adopted by our parents when he was six weeks old. He's part Navaho Indian, and when they offered to find his birth mother when he was sixteen, he told Mom that as far as he was concerned she was his mother, and we were his family, period.

He went to high school, graduated, joined the navy, served a four-year tour aboard ship in the Mediterranean and the Caribbean, missing Vietnam by some stroke of good luck. He got married when he was still in the service. He and his wife, Pat, had one child, a boy. Nineteen years later, after twelve years of being foster parents, they adopted their second child, a badly abused foster child they had cared for since he was three months old. When Jamie, their youngest, became part of our family, we felt life had come full circle: our father was adopted, Gary was adopted, and now, he had adopted a son. Jamie and our father, coincidentally, share the same birthday.

My sister married her high school sweetheart, Thomas Mindel. Her husband has been with General Motors since he graduated from high school and is a skilled trades specialist in hydraulic pipe fitting. Lolly stayed close to home, attended a local junior college, and has worked on and off for the past fifteen years as a designer and typesetter for various publishing concerns. They have two boys, Quentin, fourteen years old, and Colin, five.

My younger brother, Charles, attended college, but stopped short of graduating. For many years he has had a string of odd jobs allowing him to piece together a part-time life as a musician. He recently found a career, ironically, as a corporate head hunter, and is settling down into the struggling middle class. He still plays trombone and also sings; likes big band music, rhythm and blues, and country grunge; has gigs on occasion; and now earns enough money to pursue his second love, scuba diving. He was engaged to be married once, but broke the engagement right before the wedding. At present, he is still single.

I am the second child, went to college, delayed getting married until I was thirty, and like many women in that same life-loop, found myself, at the "height" of my career, needing to make decisions about having children. I was thirty-two when our first son was born, thirty-six when our daughter came, and forty-one when our "surprise" son arrived.

Our father, Paul Knowles, was blind since birth. He was thirteen years older than Mom. He died a few weeks after I graduated from college. Gary was married by then, Lolly was in high school, and Charles was eleven. Mom remarried a few years later to a divorcee with no children. His name was Ray Powers. Mom met Ray while continuing our father's work with Leader Dogs and the Lions Clubs International. Ray was also blind. When Mom and Ray married, Charles was the only one living at home.

For the most part, since leaving school, we have all been independent from Mom. Two of us live out of state, all of us live at least an hour's drive from her home, and we all, except Charles, have young children at home.

We are all home owners, except Charles, and all four of us live fairly simple lives. We work. We try to take good care of our children, and like hundreds of thousands of middle-class, middle-aged people today, we also take care of Mom.

Although the geographical distances are great between us, we call each other from time to time and do a credible job of keeping up with each other's lives. Since Mom has been hospitalized, we call each other more frequently, keeping tabs on what is happening with her as well as trying to knit anew a family that is no longer tied together by a powerful matriarch.

Shortly after our stepfather, Ray, died in July 1991, we struggled to gain guardianship of Mom and to come to terms with what her disease meant for our lives. When Ray died, Mom moved in with Lolly. It was the only option we had right then.

I went to Michigan to help Lolly. She was pregnant with Colin and was having trouble keeping her blood pressure under control. As a result of Ray's death, there were mountains of papers to fill out and file, and much to do. Most of all we had to decide what to do with Mom.

It was clear her mental capacities had deteriorated, and Ray's death had moved her into a new realm of dependence. In fact, it was, as each sleepless night progressed, becoming quite clear to us, unless we could find reliable, saintly, twenty-four-hour nursing service, she could never live in her own home alone again.

Along about midnight, as the song goes, Mom would be up prowling the house. She would be in an agitated state of half-sleep. In this sleep/wake state, she went from room to room turning on lights, rousing people from their sleep. Once she succeeded in waking one of us, she then asked us where she was and before we could answer, she began looking for something: a purse, some money, or Ray.

If we told her Ray died, she'd ask another question as though we hadn't said anything. We are not sure even today if she realizes he is gone.

We thought the darkness raised her anxiety, so we put a night-light in her room. When that didn't work, we bought her a big flashlight. She then made her nightly prowls with the flashlight in hand, shining the light in our eyes as she flitted from room to room.

She also had delusions. She thought there were burglars in the house. She thought Ray was trying to wake her up. She thought someone was trying to get her. Some of her delusions were sexual.

We believe the delusions began early in the spring of 1991 when Ray was in a nursing home. Unfortunately, it took us awhile to realize they were delusions.

The first clue came when she called Lolly to say Ray had been drinking. Ray, in the years we knew him, would on a rare occasion have a beer. He might have had some wilder days when he was young and in the service or single, but while he was married to Mom, we had rarely seen him with a drink in his hand, much less drunk.

It is, however, quite possible for someone to fool you. So, when the first calls came, Lolly was skeptical, but shrugged it off. Ray was in the hospital and Lolly questioned Mom about the feasibility of him getting drunk under full-time nursing care.

Mom persisted in her story and said the man in the bed next to Ray's was "slipping it to him." She also insinuated this might not be so unusual. There was a Ray, she insisted, we didn't know. None of us except Charles had lived with him, so, what she was saying was possible if not wholly plausible.

Shortly after the reported "drinking incident," Mom began accusing Ray of exposing himself to the nurses, masturbating in public, and finally, having sex with a nurse on his bed while Mom watched.

Unfortunately, the nursing staff confirmed it was Mom, not Ray, who was out of control and acting inappropriately. Ray was completely bedridden by this time and was hooked up to IVs, a colostomy bag, and occasionally some form of heart monitor. The staff was at their wit's end. Mom not only caused quite a scene by accusing the nursing staff of having sex with her husband, but she was also dangerous to Ray. She had tried on more than one occasion to unhook the IV and monitors, and to mess with the colostomy bag. They didn't want Mom visiting, but they couldn't legally ban a spouse from the ward.

She was clearly out of control. And, like many Alzheimer's victims, she was obsessed with sexual things and foul language. She not only said inappropriate things, she often disrobed or exposed herself at rather startling moments.

11

Shortly after Ray died, Lolly and I took Mom to the Turner Geriatric Clinic at the University of Michigan for testing. Mom was angry with us for taking her. She was also angry with all the doctors because they kept asking her "dumb" questions.

At one point while the doctor was testing her, trying to determine if Mom had any short- or long-term memory loss by showing her pictures, asking her questions, and having her try to duplicate puzzle patterns, he left the room for a moment. His questions and "games" agitated her beyond reason, and in a fit of pique Mom took off all her clothes and stormed out of the room shouting obscenities at the doctor.

We were sitting in the lobby waiting for her when we heard this ranting and raging woman, spitting out a string of foul words, and knew it was Mom. We looked up and there she was, with nothing on except her shoes. We called for a nurse, who grabbed a sheet from an examining room, and we wrapped her up, calmed her down, and got her dressed. Despite the craziness of her act, it did accomplish what she wanted: it ended the testing.

We had long talks with our children, who at the time ranged in age from one to ten, to explain it really wasn't okay to use the language Grandma used. We told them she was having trouble with her brain and didn't know what she was doing. We told them they were not to repeat what Grandma said, and they weren't supposed to giggle when she said bad words or did strange things.

It is not easy to explain Alzheimer's to children. For most children, there is a clear set of expectations of what a grandmother should be: she should be soft, cuddly, easy, kind, knowledgeable, loving, and fun. Their grandmother was falling apart while they watched. She periodically took off her clothes, swore, didn't know where she was, who they were or who she was, and she couldn't sit still. She was antsy, as the kids called it. She was edgy, aggressive, angry, and highly unpredictable. But, she looked, and occasionally even acted and sounded like their grandmother.

I don't know what they think or remember about those frightening times with her, but the story they always giggle over when she isn't around is the night we ordered Chinese takeout. We were all sitting at Lolly's kitchen table, passing food around, and Mom was taking some of this and some of that. We had made a big salad to go with dinner and as things were moving around the table, Mom was handed a bottle of French salad dressing. Before anyone could say anything or stop her, she opened the bottle and gleefully doused her whole plate, covering the fried rice, beef and broccoli, cashew chicken, egg roll, and stir-fried vegetables in salad dressing.

It is the least scary and least offensive thing she did then, and if it is the memory they cling to, I will be grateful.

The night wanderings were a nuisance, but were manageable. We kept the doors locked and tried gently to steer Mom back to bed, or at least to the family room to sit on the couch and look at magazines while the rest of us slept. After Colin was born, however, the situation became more complicated because Mom didn't like it when the baby cried and was always trying to "cover him up" with blankets to make him stop. Lolly moved his crib to her room so she could keep an eye on him at night and be sure Mom didn't accidentally harm him.

There were many scary aspects about keeping her in one of our homes. One day when I was making dinner, Mom came into the kitchen and picked up a piece of raw chicken and started to eat it. One of us screamed and grabbed the chicken away from her.

Mom was furious because we wouldn't let her eat it. She started screaming, saying we were horrible because we didn't want her to have anything to eat, at the same time we were struggling to get the chicken out of her hand. It was a combination wrestling-and-shouting match. We eventually got the chicken away from her and she left the room crying. It was a horrible scene, and we were badly shaken by the realization her brain could no longer differentiate between cooked and raw food, good things to eat and bad.

The kids couldn't understand what had happened and we tried to explain to them as well as to her that all we were trying to do was keep her from harming herself. The kids were scared by all the commotion. Mom was in a fury, and we knew beyond a doubt we couldn't keep her at home anymore.

Until you are faced with this decision, you cannot understand the weight it brings to your shoulders, your hands, your heart. It is one of the most difficult passages I have ever encountered. It is also tricky and treacherous, because YOU are making a life-changing decision for someone else: someone who may not agree with your decision, and, in fact, may be adamantly opposed to it.

It was not an easy decision. It was not a comfortable decision. But, it was a unanimous decision for the four siblings.

We were clear none of us had the space, lifestyle, or expertise to care for Mom at home. Three of us had small children at home, and one was single with a full-time job, part-time music career, and a dating life. Mom not only needed full-time surveillance, she needed a life with locked doors and a predictable structure. Whenever anyone, the children, neighbors, or even the UPS delivery man, came into the scene, she became agitated and volatile.

It is one thing to care for your mother but another to turn your children's lives not only upside down, but into some carefully orchestrated, no-visitors-no-loud-noises-no-slamming-doors-no-unscheduled-or-out-of-the-ordinary-comings-and-goings confinement. The situation is not sane or humane for the family or for the Alzheimer's victim.

Despite our rational, logical, loving approach to her care, we still felt guilty about not being able to care for her at home. This is, I am convinced, an unfortunate weight anyone who has cared for an Alzheimer's victim has to shoulder. I wish someone could wave a real magic wand and dissolve this guilt within us because the truth is—few individuals have the time and/or ability to do what is needed for an advanced Alzheimer's patient. The decision to seek a care solution outside the home is not only psychologically and morally heavy, it's legally complicated and expensive.

No one has been able to correctly label the legal or medical moment someone with dementia moves from making competent decisions to incompetent ones. And this, unfortunately, makes coming to the decision to put someone in a home all the more complicated.

The tricky business of Alzheimer's is that it is a disease, a raging destructive disease, that only begins to change the physical appearance of its victim in the very latest stages. You can have a full-blown case of Alzheimer's and look perfectly normal. Your temperature is normal. Your blood pressure is normal and all your blood tests are normal, but your brain is damaged beyond repair. Unfortunately, you can only see this damage in retrospect, as if the explosion is silent and the wreckage falls a heartbeat later.

In 1991, when Ray died, we had guardianship of him, but had not yet wound our way through the court system to gain legal custody of Mom. Without legal custody, we could not have access to her bank accounts, safe-deposit box, etc. Therefore, we didn't have a full picture of her financial situation.

When we were untangling Ray's estate, however, we couldn't find his life insurance policy. We searched Mom's desk. We searched the house. We looked everywhere.

When Lolly mentioned the situation to one of Mom's social workers, she suggested Lolly ask Mom about the policy. She said we should ask her every day, the same way each time, whenever Mom had a lucid moment.

So we did. After a week or more of asking her where his insurance policy was, one day she looked at us and said, "I don't know why you two girls keep asking me about Ray's life insurance. You know he was Catholic."

Catholic? We couldn't imagine what in the world being Catholic had to do with life insurance, so we asked her. Her response: "Catholics don't believe in life insurance policies, so I canceled them."

In retrospect it was funny, a great story to tell. In reality it was stunning. Without looking further, we knew it was true. We knew, in some quirky Alzheimer's moment, she had done just that: canceled both his and her life insurance policies.

We later located a notation in her records about an insurance company, and when we contacted them, they confirmed her story. The policies Mom and Ray had carried for years had been canceled without much notice. They were not cashed in, but canceled. When we tried to explain Mom was not in full control of her faculties when she did it, the officer of the insurance company who had helped us untangle what had happened, just smiled and essentially said, "tough."

I know what you're thinking. About this time you're wondering what children in their right minds would let their mother, who was so clearly out of touch, handle her own affairs.

Mom was boss. She was born boss. She lived boss. She was so good at being the boss that when you first met her, right before and even after we had gained custody of her, she walked, sat, and talked like she made sense. She seemed normal. She ran her affairs. And, if you would have given her the chance, she would have run yours.

For at least five years prior to Ray's death, and our subsequent guardianship of Mom, her "abnormalities" seemed like sporadic irrational outbursts. They did not appear to be clearly defined patterns of behavior signaling trouble. Also, her life was not without frustrations; she was struggling with a situation at home that could have driven anyone a little nuts. Ray was not well during those years, and when he was not in the hospital, she was pretty much confined at home with him. And, during this time, when we had fears about her actions, we were unable to get clear answers or help from the medical profession.

When I became the target and brunt of Mom's anger, shortly after our daughter was born in 1985, I went to see a therapist. When I told the therapist what was happening and how I felt, she told me my mother was an angry woman and I had not recognized or accepted her anger before. Her advice: cut my emotional ties with my mother and get on with my life. Again, easier said than done.

My sister and brothers and I, when we were being charitable, believed the anger and subsequent narrowing of Mom's world was not condonable, but understandable. We decided the occasional outbursts were explainable and excused by frustration, aging, and maybe a heightening of a naturally stubborn and somewhat bombastic character. Also, we had long ago learned her financial affairs were private. We did not know what they were and we knew better than to ask.

Without legal guardianship, you cannot casually assume your parent's affairs. You cannot seize their bank accounts and you cannot force them to seek professional help. In effect, even if you want to, you cannot just step in and take over. It is a complicated legal move to assume guardianship of a parent. Each state has different guidelines. And, each judge has the right to interpret these guidelines.

When Lolly went to court to gain guardianship of Ray during the spring of 1991, it seemed rather simple and straightforward. When she went, in the fall of the same year, to gain guardianship of Mom, her lawyer told her the judge she had drawn was really tough on parent/guardianship cases and she should be prepared.

Lolly was nearing the end of her pregnancy and was exhausted. When she took the stand, the judge kept her for nearly an hour, grilling her on why she wanted guardianship. Finally, nearing the end of his examination of her, he asked her what her thoughts and beliefs were about euthanasia.

The question stopped her cold. "Gosh," she said, "I haven't thought about it." The judge was silent. "I would have to give it a lot of thought," Lolly went on, not knowing what else to say but knowing we had to have guardianship of Mom, "euthanasia is a rather serious situation." The judge seemed satisfied with her answer.

Later, as Lolly was leaving the courtroom, two men in suits who had been sitting in the back of the courtroom approached her. They were two lawyers hired by the state to examine Mom and proceed, if necessary, with state guardianship. They told her they had come on their own to give Lolly support if she needed it. They knew the judge and were aware of his reluctance to grant guardianship to children. They were also aware, after talking briefly with Mom a few months earlier, hers was a clear case where guardianship was not only warranted, but the best solution. They believed granting us guardianship was preferable to the state assuming the rights. If the judge had given Lolly more trouble, they told her, they would have stepped in and testified on her behalf.

And, why would the judge in this or any guardianship hearing be reluctant to rule in the children's favor? Because of the estate. Unfortunately, there have been cases where children have asked for guardianship of an aging parent not to care for the parent, but to take control of their parent's money.

What would have happened if we had tried five years earlier to assume legal and financial responsibility for Mom and her estate? In retrospect, if we had known then what we know now, maybe we would have tried. I believe, however, because Mom was lucid then, "handled" her own affairs, and she also walked, talked, and looked "normal" most of the time, we probably would have lost. And, in losing, we would have also damaged our future credibility with the courts.

At this time there are no clear paths to take, no well-defined guidelines or even "stages" of Alzheimer's, no definitive roadmap of what to do and expect when living with Alzheimer's. Every step of the way is an experiment by trial and error: a veritable minefield of new and difficult experiences.

Alzheimer's is clearly a disease full of abnormal behaviors, but it is complex. It doesn't always take an easily recognized or neatly diagnosed path. Everyone experiences the disease differently. But, however differently it presents and progresses, the results, in the end, are the same: at some point the person can no longer care for him or herself and full guardianship must be assumed.

Once we had guardianship and understood Mom's financial situation, we were painfully aware there were no life insurance policies to fall back on. We then took a close look at what monies we had to work with and began to make a plan for what we could do to make sure she was well cared for somewhere.

There was some money in the bank and a few CDs. Our best piece of luck was probably a direct result of the early work of the Alzheimer's on her.

Because Ray had worked in the post office, he had a pretty good retirement from the government. Mom had some token income from Leader Dogs, a guide-dog agency for the blind, which was a combination of her "widow's benefits" (Dad had been the public relations director of Leader Dogs for nearly twenty years) and her own retirement benefits from the years following Dad's death when she worked as a "goodwill ambassador." Ray and Mom had also made some good investments in CDs.

In 1986, Mom realized they had feathered a rather healthy nest egg at the bank. After adding the figures together of their combined wealth, she called me one afternoon to say she was going to go to the bank and pay off her mortgage. She had ten years left on the mortgage, and paying it off would wipe out more than half of what they had put away in the bank. I tried to talk her out of it because they had a fairly low interest rate and an easy mortgage payment, even on their limited income. I also knew if something serious happened to either of them and they needed extended medical care, the only thing they had to fall back on was their savings. If she wiped out half of it, they would be in trouble.

Ray had been sick off and on by then with little things that signaled big trouble: a couple melanomas removed from his face and back, some persistent bladder problems, and an erratic heartbeat and high blood pressure. I urged her to keep her money in the bank and to keep plugging away at the mortgage.

She got angry. She told me I didn't know anything about finances and marched to the bank, withdrew the money, and paid off the mortgage.

No mortgage to pay on the house was our biggest "working" asset. It was, however, one of those good news, bad news pieces of information. The good news: it was owned free and clear. The bad news: the town Mom lived in had buyer protection laws. In order to sell the house, we would have to take care of a long list of repairs, including some rather costly ones.

For the short term, we decided not to sell the house, but to rent it and use the rental income to both upgrade the wiring, roofing, bathrooms and kitchen, and to funnel a little money toward paying for Mom's care. The longer we held onto the house, the closer we could get it up to code and ready for sale and have a little extra money to help pay for her care. It was a true fountain of wealth in an otherwise sparse financial field.

We held no delusions about the "estate." With very little discussion among the four of us, we unanimously agreed all the money should be used for Mom's care. More importantly, we would use the money to buy the best care we could find. If it took all the estate and then some, it just would.

We also decided we should hold onto the house until all other resources were exhausted. We hoped the repairs would help raise the selling price, giving us more money to spend on her care.

Our bottom line: we could afford to have Mom somewhere where she would be close to part of the family, safe, and well cared for, for as long as she needed to be there. We got lucky because the Chelsea Methodist Home had a slot for her in their small, but excellent Alzheimer's wing.

But "putting mom in a home" did not solve all the problems, nor did it neatly resolve all the issues of caring for her. We have not irresponsibly warehoused her, paid the bills, and forgotten who she is or that she is living.

She remains, for the moment, physically well while she declines mentally. It is not always clear what she needs from us. Sometimes she just needs us to sit with her. Other times she wants us to "go home before it gets dark and the roads are bad."

In contrast, our needs are complicated and troublesome. We need to have lives free from her and her suffocating disease, yet we still need to know we are somehow connected with her in spirit. We write letters she doesn't open. We visit her even though she doesn't know who we are, knowing she will not remember we came. Every time we visit we are confronted with something new and find ourselves struggling to figure out what it means. We wonder if she is in pain, if she feels any anguish looking at our faces yet not knowing who we are or why we are there. She does not like it when we call her Mom, and says her name is Ruth. If we ask her about her children, she tells us she has none.

Alzheimer's is a strange and consuming disease. It denies you the quick, clean, no-emotional-strings-attached-here's-the-nursing-home-have-a-nice-rest-of-your-life solution. We cannot turn our backs on what is happening to our mother. Lolly's life, more than the rest of ours, is occupied with Mom's day-to-day care. She is the one who negotiates with the hospital when there is a problem or Mom needs additional care. Her days are filled with papers, checks, lawyers, and reports, as well as care conferences and sewing labels in Mom's clothes. As legal guardian, Mom occupies her time and attention. For the rest of us, it occupies our thoughts, plays tricks with our emotions, and invades our waking life as well as our dreams. Even on the best of days we cannot help but wonder if Alzheimer's is hereditary, if we might not be carrying some gene or wrinkle in our brain waiting to cripple us like it has crippled Mom.

It seems like each time we tell someone about Mom we learn of someone else who is beginning to experience "trouble" with their parents. We do not feel we have as yet attained "expert status" in this realm, but find ourselves dispensing advice, listening, and hoping they will not go through what we have gone through. We pray their parent will not suffer the way ours has as she has lost her memory, her mind, her past, one little slip and tick at a time.

CHAPTER TWO

IT IS HARD TO PINPOINT THE MOMENT MOM'S ALZHEIMER'S began. Whenever the siblings get together, we try to remember what happened when. We dig further and further into the past hoping to recall some incident we can hold fast as the turning point. It is an exercise meant to bring clarity to our collective history.

Our cousin Robyn has a moment she claims as the beginning. Her mother, Aunt Geneva, one of my mother's younger sisters, is also believed to have Alzheimer's. Geneva's, however, began at an earlier age and therefore may be a different type from Mom's, which is splitting hairs in the horrible business of coping. Whether it is the early or late onset variety of Alzheimer's, once the disease progresses, the outcome is pretty much the same.

As long as I can remember, my Aunt Geneva, Robyn, Rhonda, Doug, and Brenda's mother, was never completely well. She was exhausted most of the time and looked tired and drawn. Often, she would fall asleep in the middle of a sentence; then wake ten minutes or a half an hour later and carry on as though nothing had happened.

What Robyn remembers about her mother is the fire. One day, when her mother was watching Brenda's son while she went into town to teach school, Aunt Geneva's house caught on fire. Geneva was in her late fifties at the time.

There had been a terrible storm the night before, flooding the low-water bridge in the valley where they live in the Ozarks of Missouri. Mid-morning, a neighbor, driving by, saw fire coming from Geneva's house. He knew Geneva was at Brenda's and went over to get her.

The neighbor got Geneva, and Brenda's son, and drove to her house. By then, smoke was curling up the chimney and pushing itself from beneath the closed windows and doors.

Everything Aunt Geneva owned was inside her house: antiques collected over many years, pictures from the family, pictures and possessions of Otto, her deceased husband, and everything of any worth she had ever held in her life. The neighbor went into the house and retrieved a metal file box just inside the bedroom door, but held Geneva back from going into the house afterwards because of all the smoke.

It was raining, but the rain didn't seem to touch the fire. With the bridge flooded, there was no way for the fire truck to get into the valley to put out the fire. There was no way to stop what was happening.

The neighbor tried to get her to leave, but Geneva wouldn't budge. She stood out in the rain watching the slow-burning fire darken the windows and peel the white paint from the clapboard siding. Brenda was called and came home from school. She wrapped a blanket around her mother's shoulders and took her back to her house to sleep.

For Robyn, looking back, the fire seems to be a starting point. The whole event, the fire, losing everything, then having to rebuild her home and refurnish her life, is important. The disruption the fire brought to her life, and the many decisions her mother had to make in building the new house, allowed them to see the changes resulting from the Alzheimer's more clearly and within a shorter span of time than they might have if the fire didn't occur. As Robyn explained: "She seemed fine, or at least no different than she had always been before the fire, and within a year we feared something was wrong."

For our mother the moment is less clear. We know from her checkbook and her bank accounts things were beginning to go wrong for a long time before what was happening to her became so apparent it could no longer be ignored.

Everyone I know who has struggled with a parent or friend with Alzheimer's has stories to tell. For my mother, the early stages, in retrospect, were marked by erratic emotional swings, irrational behavior, and explosions of anger.

Early Alzheimer's behavior can, at times, seem eccentric, even comical. All four of us and our families were invited to Mom's for Thanksgiving in 1985. When we arrived, we discovered her oven door had fallen off. When we asked her when it happened, she said she couldn't remember, maybe sometime back in August. When we offered to call a repairman or to go out and get the parts to fix it ourselves, she became agitated. She refused the repairs, saying there was really nothing wrong with it, and all we needed to do to cook the turkey was tie the door on. We persisted, she became angry, and in the end, we did as she said and tied the door on with a rope. Each time we basted the turkey, we had to untie the door.

Shortly after this episode, in the spring of 1986, Mom called me one day. A lifelong friend of hers had refused to run an errand for her because her friend was too busy with her own errands. My mother was furious and seemed completely out of control about the situation. When I suggested she call her friend and talk about it, she hung up the phone.

A few days later, she sent me a photocopy of a letter she wrote her friend saying she never wanted to hear from her again. The letter was pretty upsetting. I called the woman's daughter and explained I didn't think Mom meant what she had written, and added we believed Mom hadn't been herself lately. I asked her to please talk to her mother and to tell her to throw the letter away and not read it.

In retrospect, we, as her family, were irresponsible about her behavior. The story about the oven door is funny, but the one about her best friend is not. When I told someone the story about the letter Mom wrote to her friend, they looked at me in surprise and asked why I didn't immediately take my mother to a shrink.

Easier said than done. When was the last time you tried to tell your mother or father you thought they were crazy and needed psychiatric attention?

Early Alzheimer's behaviors are so erratic, so irrational, they kind of take you by surprise. Also, children are conditioned to believe their parents are right. The result of this early conditioning is to question your own sanity, not your mother's. During these early stages of Alzheimer's, we spent a lot of time trying to figure out who was right, who was wrong, and who was crazy.

We did, in fact, try several times over the next couple years to get Mom to a doctor. This rather "simple" solution is much harder to implement with an Alzheimer's victim than you can possibly imagine. First, you must remember we weren't at all sure she had Alzheimer's. After consulting with our own family doctor regarding Mom's behavior, the doctor suggested it might not be Alzheimer's, but a vitamin deficiency, the results of a small stroke, or perhaps even a brain tumor. As you can well imagine, if Mom was unwilling to talk about getting her oven door repaired, she was DEFINITELY not willing to talk about whether or not she was eating right and taking her vitamins, much less whether or not her "crazy" behavior was a result of a brain tumor.

There was nothing wrong with her as far as she was concerned. Quite the contrary, if there was anything wrong, it was with us. Any suggestion indicating we believed she might need to see a doctor brought on a terrifying avalanche of anger.

So, instead of forcing the issue and braving the anger, we waited. We waited to see if the trouble would pass. We waited to see if she would take action on her own. We wondered if she might have a vitamin deficiency. We hoped she was just in a funk or having a long string of bad days. We waited to see if she would get better. We waited to see if she would get worse. And, as Lolly once said, one of the reasons you wait so long to take action, real action, involving a clear diagnosis of Alzheimer's or any form of dementia, is knowing once the diagnosis is confirmed, you're the one left holding the bag.

It is not only true. It is complicated. The transition from functioning parent to being parented and cared for by your own children is not an easy or comfortable road.

Alzheimer's is an untested road both legally and medically. In 1994 an advisory panel on Alzheimer's from the U.S. Department of Health and Human Services, Public Health Service, National Institutes of Health, and the National Institute on Aging made a report to Congress regarding legal issues in both the care and treatment of Alzheimer's disease and related dementias. In their report they cited as one of the main difficulties of Alzheimer's, the progressive nature of the disease without clear "stages."

This lack of clear stages, and therefore clear lines and levels of impairment, make it difficult for the legal and medical profession to establish incapacity and incompetency. Several factors playing into this difficulty are noted, including: the lack of a full case history of an Alzheimer's victim because they are not capable of giving the physician or lawyer enough information to determine the level of competency before the onset of the disease, therefore physicians and lawyers cannot establish a base from which to measure decreased competency after the onset of the disease; and, "the expertise and background of the medical witness, oftentimes a family doctor who has treated the patient for years, may not reflect current knowledge of the diagnosis or treatment of Alzheimer's Disease."

It was difficult for us to make an accurate accounting and diagnosis of how Mom was doing and what was really wrong with her. In addition, it was difficult to get the medical community to listen to our concerns and take them seriously.

Our mother's doctors were her contemporaries. If we complained about Mom's occasional confusion, her memory loss, and her emotional outbursts, we were chuckled at and told by her doctors, who were experiencing some quirks of aging themselves, that these behaviors were normal for someone her age. When we insisted they weren't, we were dismissed.

You cannot just call your parents', your spouse's, or your friend's doctor and demand the doctor do something because you think these people might be ill. Nor can you call the doctor in secret after one of your parent's routine physicals and ask if the doctor possibly found anything irregular about their health or behavior. Doctors still have a strong ethical commitment to patient privacy.

We also quickly realized we couldn't force Mom to see a psychiatrist, have her physician refer her to a psychiatrist for evaluation, or get the physician to confirm our suspicions she might be crazy without her consent. During this diagnosis struggle we came to realize, once we had some official medical confirmation of what we saw as full-blown dementia, there was little a doctor could do. We had gone beyond the point where there was any glimmer of hope we might be wrong, or there was something magical or curative in a doctor's pronouncement.

During this long and difficult period from 1985 to 1990, we were becoming more and more aware Mom was no longer safe behind the wheel of a car. She clearly suffered from impaired judgment, as well as slower reflexes and a tendency to get flustered and angry when confronted with a complex series of tasks. Translation: she shouldn't drive because driving is, in fact, a complicated orchestration of hands, feet, eyes, brain, and reflexes.

The car, however, was more than transportation for Mom. It was a badge of independence as well as interdependence. When our father was alive, Mom used to drive all over the country with him, taking him from one speaking engagement for Leader Dogs to another. Every summer we would pack up the car on May 30 and "go on the road" with Dad, arriving back on September 1 for school. Mom not only drove solo during all this time, she drove, for the most part, without maps. She had an amazing mind and once she drove a route, she never forgot it. She knew every highway and shortcut from the East Coast through the Midwest. Driving was a sport, her sport, and she was clearly one of the best.

Our stepfather, like our father, was also blind, which meant, once again, Mom was the sole driver of the family. If Ray was aware of Mom's increasing inability to drive safely, he didn't let on. His lack of response or concern, however, didn't surprise us because he rarely spoke to any of us about anything. When we suggested, out of concern for both of them, that Mom should stop driving and they should start taking cabs instead, both of them got angry with us and dismissed the notion without discussion.

Despite their refusal to consider taking cabs, Lolly was getting more concerned as time rolled on. When I came to visit in the spring of 1986, Lolly suggested I go shopping with Mom so I could see for myself if she should or should not be driving anymore. I understood Lolly's desire to get some confirmation about what was going on, so I agreed and arranged a shopping trip.

At the time, Mom was sixty-six years old and was concerned about being able to pass her next driver's test coming up in the fall. It was no trouble getting her to drive because she was feeling defensive about her driving and wanted to show me how well she was doing behind the wheel for "an old bird of sixty-some."

Despite her earlier bravado, she was a little nervous as she drove and repeatedly cussed at the other motorists, who she felt had encroached on her territory. She honked her horn and shouted out the window. Other than occasionally becoming totally enraged at someone for doing something stupid and calling them a "pissant," my mother's only official oath, I never remembered her swearing in public or in private before this shopping trip. It took me by surprise, but I laughed it off, trying to defuse the situation a little. She swore at me and told me to keep my mouth shut.

While driving to the shopping mall, she saw a shoe store and stopped. It was a shoe store I had never been to before in my life. As we pulled up to the front of the store, Mom started talking about all the pairs of shoes she had bought there for me and for my brothers and sister. I was dumbfounded, first by her profanity and anger, and then by her belief we had been here before.

She insisted we go into the store. When we went inside, I told her again, I hadn't been there before. She just laughed and took my hand and told me I just didn't remember. She introduced me to the salesperson, who was equally baffled. Holding my hand while talking to the salesperson, she babbled on and on about how many shoes we had bought there and where I was living now and what I was doing. She tried to buy me a pair of shoes that weren't my size, and when I told her they wouldn't fit, she got angry.

What's happening here, you say to yourself. Who's lost it? Have I done something wrong? Have I forgotten I have been here before? Has my mother always been like this?

My head was racing, and I was beginning to feel frightened. Something was terribly wrong either with my mother, with me, or with our relationship. She didn't want to leave the store. She kept talking to the salesman and looking at soft newborn baby shoes, although no one had a little baby to buy shoes for right then. She kept finding things she wanted to buy, none of which fit her or anyone in our family. I began to realize we weren't going to be able to leave until something was purchased, so I quickly found a pair of shoes to fit me, gave the clerk my credit card, made a purchase, and got out of there.

Later on, when we had finished shopping in the mall, she started to pull out of the parking lot and became flustered. For some strange reason, she was determined she was only going to make right-hand turns. The easiest exit was a left turn, but we proceeded to make an awkward and lengthy exit to the right, circling the entire mall, then taking a long, roundabout way home because she didn't want to make any left turns.

By the time we got home, my mother sputtering and spitting with anger because I had tried to point out to her it would have been easier and shorter if we had only made a left turn or two, I was totally convinced Lolly was right: Mom shouldn't be behind the wheel of any car.

You cannot, however, get someone's license revoked because they refuse to make left-hand turns. Mom continued to drive and, to our way of thinking, get worse. By 1991, four years after the left-hand-turn incident, Lolly, realizing just how bad her judgment and reflexes had become, came up with a brilliant idea on how to get Mom's license revoked.

When it was time for Mom to get an eye exam, Lolly offered to schedule the appointment so she could take her. When she called to make the appointment, she told the doctor about her concerns and suggested he help us get Mom from behind the wheel by flunking her on the eye exam. This would have been easy for him to do since Mom had had double-cataract surgery, had poor night and peripheral vision, and it appeared, was losing vision in her left eye.

At her last exam, the same doctor had informed Mom she was legally blind in her left eye without corrective lenses.

When Mom finished her eye exam, she came into the waiting room beaming. She bragged she passed with flying colors.

As Mom was making her pronouncement, the doctor called Lolly into his office, shut the door, and began lecturing her on the fine points of growing old. He told Lolly she should be ashamed of herself even considering taking the car away from Mom. He told her young people did not understand a driver's license was a valuable piece of independence for someone growing older and it should not be taken away.

A week later, Mom was driving through town, got into an intersection, became confused, and broadsided another car. No one was hurt, but they could have been. Mom's car was damaged so extensively it had to be towed. Mom was well known in her little town both because of my father and his work with Leader Dogs, and because she ran FISH, a volunteer social service agency that interfaced with the churches, fire department, police department, and families needing help. A policeman who came to the scene of the accident recognized Mom, took her to the station, and then called Lolly to come get her.

Fortunately, Mom was completely rattled by the accident and turned over the car mess to Lolly. Lolly wisely called the insurance company, and told them as far as we were concerned the car was "totaled" and we wanted them to write us a check and take the car away.

By this time money was a major issue for Mom. She was sure she didn't have enough, and she also didn't seem to understand the difference between ten dollars and ten thousand dollars. The check from the insurance company was less than a thousand dollars. Lolly cashed it and gave it to Mom in small bills. Mom kept it in her purse and just looked at it, counting it from time to time. The idea of going out, selecting a new car, paying for it, putting gas in it, and driving it home must have seemed like a monumental task. She never mentioned it again.

Even before the car accident "crisis," we noticed she was forgetful, yet at the same time stubbornly single-minded. If she got an idea in her head, she couldn't let go of it. Often her train of thought would get tangled and if you corrected something she said or did, she'd explode.

The years preceding the crisis leading to her eventual diagnosis were emotionally complicated minefields of explosions. In the summer of 1986, when we came to visit her, she complained repeatedly about the heat. It was a very hot summer and her house had no air conditioning. In response to her complaints, my husband, Jeff, suggested she might want to think about installing central air conditioning.

She became so enraged at his suggestion she threw us out of her house saying we were not welcome there anymore. When I tried to call her from the road to make sure she was all right, she said she didn't know who I was and hung up the phone.

For the next six months, whenever I called, which I did every week just as I had all my adult life, she pretended we had a bad connection and hung up.

Ironically, despite how horrible this incident was, we were unable at the time to see it for what it was: the results of a disease. Instead, I left wondering what I had done wrong. I was emotionally drained by what happened, and struggled for years to figure out just what had gone wrong with the visit. I felt for sure, just as my sister had said at the time, I "...must have done something to piss her off."

Years later, after she had been a resident on the Alzheimer's wing at the Chelsea Methodist Home for nearly three years, Lolly and I were having a conference with the staff about Mom's care. They were expressing their concern and surprise about her recent rapid decline since she had the disease for such a short time.

We were dumbfounded to discover they dated the onset of her Alzheimer's with her testing and admission to their program. When we said no, it had been going on for years and, as far as we could judge, she had been suffering from Alzheimer's for at least ten years, they were stunned.

Incredulous, one of the staff members asked us to give them some specific examples of her behavior that might have led us to think she had Alzheimer's. When we began to tell them some of these stories, they agreed but were still surprised.

"If you've been dealing with this for ten years," one of them said, "you must be nearly burned out."

Unfortunately, all too many family members today find themselves struggling with years of erratic behavior before something tragic or undeniably crazy happens that cannot be laughed off or ignored.

Memory loss is not legally or medically recognized as being equal to impaired judgment. Memory loss as a result of Alzheimer's, in our experience, however, does not occur in isolation. The memory loss is jumbled with erratic behavior in such a way it becomes difficult to determine what came first: the erratic behavior or the memory loss. The two seem to feed on each other in such a frenzied manner they can sometimes produce dizzying results.

Because there are no clear outlined "stages" to watch for, family members are left living through the complexities true short-term memory loss can cause, wondering what is going to happen next. When memory loss blooms forth into erratic behavior, family members are left with the complicated task of measuring this behavior with some "true" erratic behavior in context of a person's history, both recent and past.

The inherent difficulties of sorting out and pinpointing when someone's behavior shifts from eccentric to erratic complicates and clouds the issues at hand: i.e., the real difference between forgetfulness and memory loss, and the fine borderline between competency and incompetency. Self-doubt regarding your own suspicions coupled with a lack of clear guidelines from the medical and legal establishment make it difficult for a family member to know when to "push the issue" and begin assuming the role of parent to their parent.

The same advisory panel that recognized the difficulty of identifying competency for Alzheimer's victims also concluded "...a person in the early stages of Alzheimer's disease retains the legal right to make his or her own decisions absent a court finding of incapacity and may well have the current ability to establish voluntary delegations of decision making."

This conclusion is chilling. I do not know anymore when Mom was truly competent and in her "right mind." I suspect it was many years ago. During the years preceding the "beginning," we now suspect there were "normal" moments and "abnormal" moments in her thought processes. Also, we suspect there were times in the beginning of her decline when she had clear blinding moments of rational thought.

Our father was blind from birth. There had been some instrument damage to his eyes during his delivery. In addition, he was premature and was kept in an incubator in which they pumped too much oxygen, causing further damage. He had "pinhole" vision. There were one or two optic receptors in one eye that continued to function, but he couldn't really see anything. Ray, on the other hand, lost his sight as an adult from a degenerative retinal disease. On rare occasions, he would wake up in the morning and for ten seconds or less, when he first opened his eyes, he could see clearly. It was a very painful and disturbing event for him. It caused him a great deal of anguish because it made him think for a moment he might, if the doctors only knew what to do, be able to see again. He was grateful for these brief moments of sight, but yet, knowing they would end just as quickly as they came and there was nothing anyone could do to bring his vision back to him permanently, he wished with all his heart these vision explosions would cease to happen.

I imagine the rare moment or two of clarity in her years of confusion must have elicited a similar response for my mother. Once, when I was visiting her at the Chelsea Methodist Home in 1994, we were walking down the hall together. All around us were people shuffling about in walkers, bumping against the walls, and talking to themselves. It was a typical day on her floor. Mom, like the other patients, was doing her own version of cruising and mumbling, struggling to get a string of words to stay together. All of a sudden, she grabbed my hand and started to giggle. With her other hand, she made a gentle sweeping arch, as if to say: see what we have here. "You know," she said, pulling me closer to her in order to whisper in my ear, "sometimes I say to myself, Ruth, you really must be crazy to be here." Then she giggled again and slipped back into her other world where words and thoughts get tangled and lost.

It is difficult for us to think back over the years, to piece together the past and where it began to fall apart. But, it is nothing compared to trying to think about what it must have been like for her, waking some mornings able to "see" for a terrible teasing moment some piece of her mind and her memory she had lost in the night.

Chapter Three

November 1992

WE ARE TAKING THE TWENTY-TWO-HOUR TRAIN RIDE FROM Raleigh, North Carolina, to Ann Arbor, Michigan, to have Thanksgiving with Mom, but we cannot tell her we are coming. My brother will drive a double shift on his truck route so he can take a three-hour nap, put his son and his wife in his pickup and drive all night from Paducah, Kentucky, to Michigan to come too.

We're lucky, Mom is living in one of the best Alzheimer's units in the country and she's happy. She doesn't know she's there. She thinks she has a beautiful new house. She thinks the people living across the hall from her really live down the street. She used to think she worked at the Chelsea Methodist Home.

41

Now she tells us she pitches in only when her neighbors need help or when there's a party or some special event. If we were to tell her we were coming, she would go immediately to the elevator to wait for us, not knowing day from night, Thanksgiving from New Year's Eve.

Time and space mean nothing to her. Last Christmas, we gave her one of those programmable telephones. We installed all our numbers into the memory so all she had to do was push one button to call each of us long distance. We even labeled the buttons. She called me a couple times a day asking me to bring her some bologna and a loaf of bread. When I tried to explain I couldn't because I lived in North Carolina, she got angry because I wouldn't do what she wanted. She doesn't call any of us anymore. She has forgotten how to use her fancy phone.

We are coming to Lolly's house for Thanksgiving because we are going to throw a wedding reception for our youngest brother, Charles. He isn't getting married until next July, but the staff at the Methodist Home has asked us to be a little "creative" about the wedding. July is too far away. Mom is obsessed with his upcoming marriage and is becoming agitated. Also, it is unclear what she will know or remember by next July. We all agree it would be nice for her to believe that he is, at last, married.

Since Lolly has the role of legal guardian she sees Mom the most. She also lives in Chelsea. A lucky break for Mom and the rest of us; a burden for Lolly. I worry about Lolly more than I do about Mom. Mom is fine. She's happy, well fed, safe, and feels independent and productive. Lolly, on the other hand, understands what is happening.

Alzheimer's is a cruel disease. It sneaks up on you. Little things go wrong at first. So little, you can easily push them out of your mind: a forgotten appointment, misplaced handbag, a garbled sentence, a burst of anger or frustration, or the nagging fear there may not be enough money for you to live on. It is as though the fringes of Alzheimer's border on reality, better still, that this fringe is just the reality of aging.

Full-blown Alzheimer's is frightening. Reality becomes distorted. Up and down, true and false, even life and death get confused because at some crucial point, everyone who has a loved one with Alzheimer's understands that the person they once loved is gone. They are, although still breathing, in fact, dead and will never return again.

The brain is a complex and mysterious machine. Alzheimer's is usually positively diagnosed only by autopsy: by the pattern of destruction in the brain. After intensive testing at the Turner Geriatric Clinic of the University of Michigan Medical School, we were told Mom was a textbook case: she had no short-term memory and exhibited several other classic Alzheimer's symptoms.

Ironically, Alzheimer's victims often cannot recognize their primary caregiver. Such was the case with Mom. When I would call to talk to Mom while she lived with Lolly, she would tell me all about the wonderful people she was staying with although she couldn't identify who they were or where she was living. Once we moved her to the Methodist Home, she was able to remember my sister's name and identify Lolly's children as her grandchildren.

You can laugh about something like that, but it's confusing. It feels bad and your feelings get hurt although your head tells you it's just the disease doing its damage.

If you're the "good kid," the one who calls every Sunday, the one who takes on the responsibility of being the guardian, the one who sends flowers on Mother's Day and tries to do the right thing, Alzheimer's can drive you crazy. The only way to be the happy survivor of an Alzheimer's victim is to lie, and the "good kid" would never lie to her mother.

That's how we survive. We lie. It's not an easy thing to do. It feels wrong. It feels like you're living dangerously, because if you get caught, your mother is going to kill you.

Like sins, there are lies of commission and lies of omission. Our first lie for Thanksgiving is not telling Mom we're all coming. Our second is telling her the reason Charles and his fiancee aren't eating Thanksgiving dinner with us is because they have flown to Las Vegas to get married: the only way Charles could get Friday off from work in order to attend his wedding reception was to work Thanksgiving.

We think the lie about Las Vegas is a great lie. We rehearse it a little and tell all the kids. When you're into lying, you've got to make sure all your bases are covered. Once we've got the lie down pat, we've got to decide who is going to deliver it.

Nobody volunteers. Timing is everything when you're telling lies to an Alzheimer's victim. You've got to wait for the lucid moment, the little crack in the window of reality, the few heartbeats where she's with you all the way. Otherwise you've got to repeat yourself, and anyone who's ever told a lie knows repeating the lie is the best way to get caught.

It's my turn. Mom is in Lolly's kitchen. The table is set for turkey and all the fixings. We're standing around trying to take a reading on how the afternoon is going to roll. It's clear Mom doesn't know it's Thanksgiving. She hasn't called anyone by their correct name or any name, which is usually a bad sign. You can see the little kids are making her nervous.

"Where's Charlie?" she asks, clutching her purse in her hands, looking around the room trying to get her bearings.

There is this terrible silence. I haven't felt like this since I was ten. Nobody says anything. Gary, the oldest, looks down at his shoes.

"You're not going to believe this," I tell her, looking at my siblings for support, "but he called this morning. He and Donna are in Las Vegas. They're getting married."

"I just had a feeling," she says, and we all breathe a little easier because we know she got it, "they were going to do that."

"Aren't you glad," the guilt of the lie breaks over me like a wave about to knock me off my feet. "She's a real nice woman. I think Charlie's lucky, don't you?"

"I just had a feeling," she says again. And Gary straightens his glasses and moves into the kitchen to help Lolly carve the turkey. The deed is done.

I trust Lolly's instincts since she is the one who has the most contact with Mom. She's the one who is going to be left taking care of her after the rest of us pack up and go home. She's ordered the cake and talked to the nursing staff and made the arrangements for the reception to be on the Alzheimer's wing.

Lolly says it's the only way the thing is going to work. It has to be on the Alzheimer's wing because Mom is at her best there. It's where we stand the greatest chance of her remembering. If Lolly says we're having cake and punch and fake wedding pictures on the Alzheimer's wing, then that's what we're doing and I'm willing to back her one hundred percent.

Charles doesn't want to do it. He knows it's the "right thing," but he doesn't want to have to spend any time with all those people who have Alzheimer's. It's creepy. It brings it all too sharply into focus. Charles wants us to have the cake and the pictures at Lolly's house.

Gary isn't the kind of person to buck the crowd, he never has been. Still he brings up the question one more time trying to be sure we should go through with this.

Lolly looks at me and I tell Gary I think Lolly's right. It has to be at the Alzheimer's wing. He nods his head and I know he'll be there.

Charles will too. We've had to use him for a lot of things in the past couple of years. For the moment, he's the one Mom responds to, so he was the one who drew the short straw to take her to the Methodist Home the first time.

Lolly and I set it up, but when the time came for Mom to go, it was Charles who took her. It was Charles who told her what a neat place it was, it was Charles who sold her on the idea.

Charles has also been the beneficiary. He manages to catch all the credit. Mom believes Charles bought her a new bed, although Lolly bought it and Tom, her husband, delivered it and set it up. The fancy spread and headboard came with a birthday card signed from the four of us, but Charles was the only name she remembered.

Like con artists setting someone up for the sting, we have begun to act like gangsters with Charles as the mouthpiece.

About six months ago, Lolly, who had just returned from spending an afternoon cleaning Mom's house and painting her garage so we could rent it in order to help pay for the bills at the Methodist Home, called me in a fit. Mom had called her and told her she only had one child, Charlie. We both laughed about it and decided if Charles was an only child, and if we knew for certain we had siblings, then he couldn't possibly be ours. And if he wasn't ours anymore, then we were no longer responsible for him.

We give Charles a hard time. We all laugh about the only child business. It's even funnier since Gary used to claim he wanted to be an only child when he grew up.

We drink a toast to Charles and his new bride before we carve into the turkey. Mom looks a little bewildered and we all start talking again about how good Donna is and what a surprise it was they called to say they were going to Las Vegas to get married.

The phone rings. Lolly gets up to answer it and we all know it's Charles checking to see if the rest of us have arrived. She's great on the phone and manages to chat her way through the conversation as though she's talking to a neighbor, which is what she tells Mom when she hangs up.

There's a lot of food on the table and it's getting passed around and we all sense the confusion Mom feels. It has been more than a year since she could correctly identify a fork from a spoon. Food is complicated. She's not sure what to do with the gravy so she passes it on. She makes a mess of things, putting mashed potatoes on her salad plate, cranberry sauce on her green beans, and generally blowing the conventional wisdom of turkey and dressing, gravy and sauce.

The older kids giggle but stifle it in a hurry as the rest of us turn on the ice-from-hell look. The kids make Mom nervous. Most of the time they're fairly sensitive to her needs. They know, however, if they do the same thing she has just done, they will be sent from the table. The situation is funny, yet filled with tension.

Someone makes a joke and we all laugh. I concentrate on eating the dressing. It's the best yet and

I want to remember the good of the day: we're all here, and Mom's alive and physically well and happy. It's hard, because the truth is, her disease has taken a toll on us all.

It's a gray day outside. My kids swear they've seen some snow flurries so we all squint our eyes and try to see what they want to see. If we look real hard at one place for a long time, we can see a flake or two.

Mom is tired. She starts asking about how she's going to get home. She wants to know who is going to take her. The boys get elected. For some reason she does better with the men, maybe she trusts them more or maybe she doesn't think she can question their judgment. One time when Lolly and I took her back after having her over to the house for a long day last fall, Mom fell apart. She didn't recognize her room, the Alzheimer's wing, her fellow residents, anything. She became frightened and began screaming that she wanted to go home. She said we tricked her. It scared the kids to death. Since then we're more careful about who picks her up and who takes her back and we try not to have the kids in tow on the return.

She believes she has lost her jacket. We know she left it in her room and try to reassure her it will be there. Next, she's sure we've switched purses on her, which we haven't, and keep showing her the purse and reassuring her it is hers. Her name is written all over it in ballpoint pen. A few months ago she signed her name on everything she could find. Her purse almost looks as though it has been purposely stamped with the design of her name, like a designer fabric. She studies the writing on her purse as though she doesn't recognize her signature or is unsure of what it says. No one says anything. We've learned not to push, to let her come to some resolution on her own. We do not want to agitate her.

"It's getting dark and I've got to get going, I left the house empty. There's no one there. I shouldn't be gone for long," she says, then she accepts our hugs and kisses and heads out with Tom, Gary, and Jeff as though she is being escorted by a bevy of bodyguards.

"Not a good day," Lolly says as she heads back to the kitchen to clean up, "let's hope tomorrow is better."

We all agree.

Charles calls to say he and Donna are running a little behind schedule and we make plans to meet at the Methodist Home. Gary's running late, too, but manages to pull up just as we're packing the kids into the car. Pat and Jamie, his wife and son, won't be coming because they've decided to spend the day with Pat's sister. Nobody thinks this will present a problem since Mom couldn't make an accurate head count on the best of days anymore.

We swing by the bakery to get the cake. It looks great: pale yellow roses and white bric-a-brac around the edges and a big green frosting "Congratulations Charles and Donna" emblazoned down the middle of a field of flowers and wedding bells. It's every kids' dream-fix of butter-cream frosting.

Donna and Charles are waiting for us in the lobby when we arrive. My stomach jumps and flops and jitters. We could get caught, a little voice screams in my head. She could be having a bad day. This whole thing could backfire.

Mom is in the television room watching Star Trek when we arrive. One of the staff sees the huge cake and realizes there's been a little miscommunication. The reception was supposed to be their dessert today, but somehow the message didn't get quite far enough and they've just eaten pie with their lunch. The staff member touches my arm and suggests we give them time to "walk it off" a little. My stomach knots up. I'm afraid our plan will fail, but I smile back and say it's no problem because we'll need a little time to set up.

Mom pulls Charles aside and tells him no one came to get her for Thanksgiving. She tells him she didn't have turkey, in fact, she didn't get anything to eat all day. She tells him we've all abandoned her. Charles tries to reassure her we did come, she did eat with us, she just forgot. She shakes her head no.

The subject gets changed and we all start talking about the wedding. Donna shows off her ring. She looks pretty, dressed in creamy white slacks and a beautiful white sweater with sequins and little seed pearls. She's being an incredible sport. Jeff starts taking pictures.

That's the key: pictures. One of the staff comes up and asks what are we going to do if she doesn't remember. We tell her we're taking pictures, lots of pictures. We plan to send them to her as soon as they're developed so she can look at them and the staff can talk about them with her. We decide it would help if there were pictures not only of the family and her friends, but also pictures of Mom and the staff with Donna and Charles.

The nurse nods her head and goes to tell the rest of the staff. One by one they show up and stand with Mom so we can take pictures with the cake and the smiling bride and groom.

The other residents begin to wander into the room. Donna and Charles cut the cake. We tell everyone it's a wedding reception for Ruth's youngest son and ask them if they want punch and cake. They want to know who Ruth is, who the son is, who we all are, so we smile and usher them to tables and cut cake, talk, pour punch, and smile.

The kids are having a great time. The residents love having them around. The kids aren't afraid and go from table to table and eat cake, refill punch cups, and talk.

One of the ladies keeps wrapping her cake in her napkin and putting it in her lap and telling the other ladies at her table she hasn't gotten any cake yet. There is a bit of commotion over the "unserved" woman and we don't know quite what to do, so we cut her another piece.

One thing leads to another and pretty soon, the woman with the short memory about the cake has four or five pieces of cake tightly wrapped in our decorative little wedding napkins all piled in her lap. We switch to serving her punch and let her build up a line of punch cups.

Another woman finishes her cake and folds her napkin. Once it is folded she tears it into strips then takes her neighbor's napkin and does the same thing. She works her way around the room, from table to table, folding and tearing napkins until she has a stack of torn napkins nearly two inches thick. No one seems to mind.

We sit and talk with the residents, answering questions, over and over again. Many of them have lost their natural affect and seem flat, or smile when they are saying something angry or sad. It is the same with Mom. Words and actions no longer match: interaction is confusing on both sides. In the chaos of the moment we can see what kind of people all these confused folks once were, and can imagine how lively and competent they must have been before the disease took hold. Many of the women on the wing with Mom used to be teachers and nurses. They, like Mom, all have neatly cut and curled hair and wear "good" clothing. You have a sense they led "sensible" lives, kept clean houses, raised children, grew beautiful gardens, had friends, threw parties, had hobbies, volunteered. The loss is overwhelming.

The cake is nearly gone. Everyone has eaten their sugar roses. People begin to wander back to watch television or walk the halls. The staff works hard to bring people by to say hello and have their picture taken with Mom.

Mom starts saying it is getting dark. It is her way of telling us we need to go. She doesn't like being out when it is dark and she doesn't want us to have trouble on the roads. It is not quite three o'clock in the afternoon.

We clean up and prepare to say our good-byes. Mom wants to show us her house. She wants us to see the changes she's made. Her room is the same as it has been since she moved in over a year ago, but we all ooh and aah over the improvements she's made. She tells us she only uses this part of the house now and has closed off the rest of it because she doesn't need it anymore. The walls of her room are covered with colored pictures and cut-and-paste artwork she has done in her therapy group. It looks like the work of a young child. She has several bouquets of silk flowers near her window. She waters them daily. She says she can't believe how long they've lasted.

She can't find her purse and gets confused because our coats are in her closet. The purse is on her desk and we point out where she has written her name on it again. She takes the purse and holds it as though we might try to take it away from her.

One of the staff members follows us down the hall so she can unlock the elevator. Mom stands back to say her good-byes. She never goes near the elevator. One man does on occasion and when he becomes fixated about the elevator, they put a library table in front of it so you have to move the furniture when you come and go.

When we get back to Lolly's, we all just sit around and talk. Mom liked the reception and all the attention. The cake was beautiful. We are all exhausted.

Lolly tells us two people died on the Alzheimer's wing last week. There's silence. We had all believed as long as Mom was on the Alzheimer's wing, she was safe. When the disease progressed to the point where it could kill her, we thought she would be moved to a total nursing care unit. We have been living with a false hope that her continued residency on her little happy hall meant she was doing fine, and nothing could harm her.

Charles says he's read about some new medication, some experimental drug believed to reverse the Alzheimer's process. It is a sobering thought: to go backward. We have been through so much unraveling and so much grieving, to go backward, to day by day reverse this terrible process, to experience all the hurt, confusion and anger, feels akin to walking through Hell again. We are reminded of Edgar Allen Poe's *The Monkey's Paw*, where the family wishes for their son to return from the grave only to be stalked by his decayed and disfigured body.

We've all read the books. We know about the damage done to our mother's brain. Can this drug reknit the brain? If it can, can it do it overnight? Or is the repair as tedious and drawn out as the damage has been?

Gary shakes his head, "It's just too hard to think about," he says, his voice flat as though he is speaking about the death of a friend. "She was always the boss. I mean, ALWAYS the boss. Now she's like this."

He doesn't need to go on because we know we've crossed over some invisible line no miracle drug can touch. Mom's gone and in some quiet and horrible way we all feel quite alone.

Charles and Donna have spent the night and the kids get up early to have their "Christmas" breakfast. It is the Saturday after Thanksgiving and we've decided since we are all together, we'll have our family Christmas.

When I get out of the shower, Lolly is in the kitchen scrambling eggs.

"Mom's had two bad days," she says, cracking eggs, "what would you think about having our Christmas, then going to get her for lunch and after lunch letting her open her presents?"

There are six kids upstairs rattling presents under the tree. It feels like a Christmas morning. There is a lot of excitement and anticipation in the air. It's another lie, a double lie: Christmas when it's not Christmas and a not-Christmas without her. But, Lolly's right. The chaos and confusion would throw Mom. We stand a chance of making it work if it is controlled, if all the action and excitement is centered on her.

Last Christmas, the real Christmas, was a disaster. She didn't understand what we were doing with all the packages. She didn't know what presents were hers and kept giving them back and putting other things, stuffed toys and candy and Christmas ornaments, in her bag. She got angry when we took the kids' things away from her and was sullen and agitated during dinner. We are not anxious for a repeat.

"I don't like it," I tell Lolly and she nods her head, "but you're right."

Mom's had some good days over the last couple months, where she's recognized Lolly, made appropriate responses, and generally seemed on top of things. One day, she even noticed Lolly had gotten a haircut and commented on how nice it looked. That night Lolly called me to say it was strange, almost as though she was better, that she was herself again.

We open our presents, clean up, then send Gary and Tom to go get her. They take his pickup truck. Cole, our youngest, wants to go too. He loves Gary's big truck. We promise him a ride some other time. It is funny to think of Mom jostling along sandwiched between Tom and Gary, coming to a Christmas that isn't Christmas that she probably won't remember.

Mom doesn't remember much about yesterday or the wedding. We kid Charles about being the only child, but tread lightly on the reality that Mom doesn't know the rest of us are her children. When Mom's sister, Jessie, came to visit a few months ago, Mom told her Gary had died a long time ago. Gary is half Navajo. He was adopted when he was an infant. The rest of us are "naturals" and are a fiery blend of Scotch stubbornness and Irish fight. He has the classic American Indian disposition. He is slow to anger. He can't drink worth a damn. He's quiet and he is our brother to the bone. We cannot joke about Mom thinking he's dead.

No one says anything, but Gary senses she does not know him. He has this great idea about getting a picture of Mom with the four of us while we are together today, then we should all get portraits done of our various families and put the pictures together in a collage so she can see who belongs to whom. Oddly enough, she can correctly identify all of our children as her grandchildren. She can even call Hedy, my daughter, the only granddaughter, by name. She cannot, however, positively identify the rest of us as belonging to her.

She is clearly confused by all the people in Lolly's house. She doesn't let go of her purse. She keeps showing me the three brass dots decorating the front flap of her purse and tells me she knows the purse is hers because it has those dots. She ignores the fact that her name is written all over the tan vinyl surface. Her fingers trace the dots as though she is reading braille.

One by one the kids come into the family room to sit with her. They watch television together and cuddle. She is responsive to them. Charles sits with her and talks about the wedding. I mend a hole in the sleeve of her coat and tack down the loose interfacing.

It is her favorite jacket and she has adorned the lapels with a dozen or more Lions Club pins. Our father was active in Lions Clubs International and she collected the pins over thirty years of traveling with him. When she talks about Dad, her voice is a little distant and slightly strained as though she is trying to remember him. She tries to give away one of Lolly's favorite childhood dolls to Hedy. Lolly intervenes saying it was the last doll Dad gave her and Mom looks a little puzzled. "Yes," she says, looking at the doll and straightening its yellow braids, "Paul was your father."

Dinner is a hodgepodge of leftover Thanksgiving. We eat heartily and laugh a lot. We talk about Donna and Charles' wedding and the reception at the Methodist Home. Mom seems to be following the conversation and gives her approval or nods when something is said to her. She says she thinks Jessie is coming. We tell her she isn't. She doesn't believe us and keeps saying you can never tell what will happen. She says she just has a feeling Jessie might show up for dinner.

Mom has always had feelings and a strong intuition. It is hard to keep from crying or screaming because although her head is scrambled, her heart is strong. She is strong, as strong and as stubborn as an ox and would probably live forever if her brain weren't dying.

We clear the dishes and send the kids upstairs to get her Christmas presents. We explain that although it isn't Christmas, Gary and I won't be able to come back up until next summer so we want to give her our gifts now. "Whatever you want," she says and shakes her head a little, "I know you can't come."

Donna and Charles give her a beautiful framed wedding portrait. It is not their wedding picture exactly, but a picture taken of them at a friend's wedding: Donna was a bridesmaid and Charles is in a tuxedo. It's a great picture and a nice touch. We tell her we'll hang it today when we take her home. She keeps saying how lovely it is and calling Charles to see it. She tries to give it to him as a gift and he gives it back. She tries again and eventually Charles gets the hint and leaves the room as Donna gives it back to her a fourth time and tells her it is for her, for her house. It is a gift from them to her.

She doesn't get it. She puts the picture back in the box and asks Lolly if she wants it. Tom gets a picture hanger and a hammer and lays them near the picture and tells her he'll hang it up in her house when he takes her home. We talk a little about where it might look nice. She's not sure so we talk a little about her new house and about all the lovely things she has there.

I get a fancy shopping bag with a Christmas scene on it and nice handles and put the hammer and picture in it. We give her another present.

There are several boxes of candy. Mom has developed a sweet tooth. She likes candy and likes having it around to share with her friends. There are lots of little things, a half dozen or so small packages for her to open: some new cotton socks, a gaudy plastic necklace she loves and puts on immediately with the other two necklaces she's wearing, and a small red change purse with a key ring the kids picked out for her.

She likes the change purse and her face brightens in a way we haven't seen it brighten in a couple years. The kids show her how it zips and closes and how she can put her keys on the ring. She works the zipper and snaps the snap and asks for her purse so she can get something to put in it. When she opens her purse, it is full of small plastic juice cups from the Methodist Home and she tries to give one to each of the kids. They are gracious and take them, then give them back, knowing they belong to the home and she should return them. She gathers them up and stacks them so they'll fit snugly in her bag. She holds the change purse and smiles. It's a great gift.

Three Christmases ago, before we were able to accept or understand what was happening to her, she stood up in the middle of dinner to make an announcement. It was quite uncharacteristic of her and was done with such pomp and ceremony, it took us by surprise. She had been edgy all that morning and held onto her purse all day, clicking the tight brass latch open and shut with a nervous kind of tick.

She tapped on the edge of her glass and called for our attention, then took a used envelope out of her purse and began her announcement. I don't remember her hands shaking, but thought her voice seemed strange, flat and distant and distressed. She talked for a few minutes without making much sense, our stepfather quiet by her side as though the speech had been rehearsed, then she called us one by one to stand up, then she handed out money.

It was a strange gesture, one she had never done before or since. We were all a little uncomfortable, but took the crisp bills as directed and took our seats. When the envelope was empty, she sat down and continued with her meal as though nothing had happened.

I carried the money in my purse for almost a year before I spent it, searching for something that reminded me of her. It was the last gift she gave any of us.

We have put all her presents in her pretty bag and have reassured her Tom will hang the picture as soon as he takes her home today. She says it's late and she wants to go now. We ask her if she wants to stay for dessert.

Yes, dessert. She likes dessert and says she'll stay. Gary tells her we want to get a picture of her with her kids and she startles as though he's said something odd.

"I have no kids here," she says, looking around the room, "no kids. I had no kids. No, I had one kid. Only one child. That one there." Then she points to Charles and walks toward him to hug him. "This is my child," she says, "my only child."

"Oh, Mom," we kid her, "come on, we're your kids too."

"No," she says shaking her head, "no, I only had one kid. This one, but you," she says, pointing to Lolly, "you look a lot like the Barrs. You could be one of Grace's kids."

We try to laugh and all crowd around her, our arms fumbling to link with hers, to draw us all close together. Jeff struggles to get us all in the picture, to get us all in focus.

"Okay, you guys," he calls out, "smile."

CHAPTER FOUR

APRIL 1994

IT IS TEN O'CLOCK ON A WEDNESDAY EVENING. I HAVE
just finished conducting a workshop for the winners
of the Raleigh Fine Arts Society's high school short
story contest. A handful of parents and students have
stayed past the workshop to talk and ask for encour-
agement. When the others at last leave, one lone
parent takes me off into a corner and tells me her
son is good, really good, but he writes bloody stories,
stories she believes we wouldn't accept in this contest.

She wants me to help him. She quickly adds she
does not want me to teach him. She does not believe
he needs help with his writing. She thinks his stories
are good and he should continue to write the way he
writes. What she wants me to do is help him find a

place in this community where his writing will be accepted. She wants me to make some connection in my world for her son.

I give her some suggestions of places he might turn to, people who might be able to help him, but I do not offer to become his mentor. I do not know much about science fiction nor am I hooked into the science fiction writing/publishing network.

Her desire, however, for her son to find a comfortable and nurturing place for himself strikes a chord with me. As I pull out of the parking lot, too tired to remember clearly if I need to turn left or right to go home, I think about my mother.

My oldest brother, Gary, drove up from Kentucky to see Mom last weekend. He spent three hours with her one afternoon and during all that time, she was unable to make a connection with him—who he was, who she was, who they were together. Later, Mom got angry when my sister, Lolly, whom Mom didn't recognize either, had to leave. When Lolly was telling Mom it was time for her to leave, an attendant happened by and asked if Mom would like the cup she was carrying refilled. My mother, angered and confused, and missing the connection between her cup and the man's question, threw the water she had been drinking at him.

My sister sounded tired on the phone when she told the story: tired and drained and aggravated. For the last few years every family visit and every holiday has been severely touched and even damaged by our mother's illness. It is the first time I have heard Lolly complain or feel resentful, but what she says is the truth: the specter of our mother and her illness have moved across our lives like a shadow we can't shake.

For one clear moment, easing into the string of headlights going home from the high school workshop, I understand what is happening to our family: we have let go of any chance for a miracle.

Our family has lived by miracles. In 1954, the year Lolly was born, our father was diagnosed with throat cancer. He was not supposed to live. No one with cancer lived back then. But then the first miracle came: radiation treatments.

He was one of the first people in the United States to receive radiation treatments. They were given to him on an experimental basis at the University of Michigan. As experiments go, it wasn't a bad one. Unfortunately, they overestimated how much radiation was needed to cure the disease and managed to damage two-thirds of his lungs in the process, but they made a miracle and he lived.

Thirteen years and many miracles later, having developed diabetes and undergone another lifesaving innovation of modern medicine, a pacemaker, he died of a massive brain tumor. Still, at no time during his life of illness had we ever let go of the hope of a miracle. We had kept clear of the shadows.

It is hard to hope for miracles with Alzheimer's. Unlike cancer, heart disease, or even AIDS, there are no "good days" where a remission steps in and the patient is given a brief window of normal. There are no miracles. In fact, given the phenomenal destruction to the brain, it is hard to envision what a remission would be like. There is no phase of the disease you would like to have anyone you know stuck in or returned to because of some medical miracle. There is no remotely satisfactory half-life a miracle might bring.

In fact, the idea of such a "remission" is terrifying. It makes my stomach hurt to think of my mother caught in a moment in which her memory is returned and she knows my name, her name, her past, her present, her grandchildren's names, and is confronted by the staggering sadness of all that she has lost.

The damage done to her brain has robbed her of her connection with the world. She has lost her past, her future, her place in time.

There have been all too many moments over the past few years, as Lolly, Gary, our younger brother, Charles, and I have talked about some incident, some outburst, some new loss she has experienced, when we have stopped and almost simultaneously said: "She isn't really Mom."

Families living with Alzheimer's need more than a big-time medical miracle. We need a way to sort out just how all of us are connected in the world. We need a way to keep ourselves tied together. It is more than flesh and blood. It is history. It is past and promise. It is the shared secrets between people who have known each other for a lifetime.

Although the "warning signs" of Alzheimer's read like a checklist for aging, it is more than just an intense version of aging. Yes, when you age, your memory gets fuzzy, little details of events blur together, and you sometimes jumble the past and the present. As you age, or just find yourself pushed by the staggering demands of life, you can sometimes forget where you're going or what you're supposed to be doing. But, your mind is not a total blank and you have emotions.

Alzheimer's takes all that away. Mom still has emotions, but they are often inappropriate or wildly out of control. The best description of Alzheimer's was given to us by one of the doctors who tested Mom. After describing Mom as a "textbook case," he suggested we tell our children: "When grandma goes to sleep, the tape recorder in her head, the one recording everything she sees, hears or thinks, accidentally gets erased along with a little bit of the past." With Alzheimer's there is no day in the future that will ever be as good as the day you just erased.

And, while Alzheimer's is erasing the past, it erases the present, jumbles language, and makes a mess of emotions. It has been a long time since my mother's face showed joy, surprise, recognition, or expectation. It has been a long, long time since any of us have heard her laugh.

And while Alzheimer's is messing with the memory and emotions, it does some interesting things along the way. Earlier in our mother's illness, when she was first moved to the Alzheimer's wing at the Chelsea Methodist Home, the staff took away her cigarettes for safety reasons. They told her they would keep the cigarettes for her in the nurses' office and she could come down there anytime she wanted to smoke.

Even though the tobacco industry claims nicotine is not addictive, our mother tried all her life to quit smoking but was never successful. Even when our father was diagnosed with terminal throat and lung cancer, clearly linked to his smoking, she was unable to quit and continued to smoke in the backyard and in secret the rest of her life. In fact, in the years preceding her hospitalization for Alzheimer's, she probably smoked two to two and a half packs a day.

Once the cigarettes were removed from her purse, however, she forgot she smoked, and within a day or two quit going to the nurses' station.

She has also forgotten on occasion what her false teeth were for, and has discarded her glasses because she forgot they were hers. She is extremely nearsighted and probably can't see two feet in front of her without them.

The cigarettes, teeth, and glasses don't really matter. They are the symptoms. They are visual manifestations of the trouble inside. They are not the things we struggle with when we think about her.

We are like the mother who pulled me aside at the short story contest to whisper her concerns. We want to find a connection. We are looking for something or someone who can "hook our mother up" to this life, our lives, this world again. We watch anxiously for a sign that this person who looks like our mother really IS our mother. We are looking for a reason to be grabbing for miracles.

Instead, we are gasping for air as we drown along with her in the dark sea of her never-ending illness. I have quit telling funny stories to our children about what grandma was like before she became ill because that time is too far gone for me to pull it back again. It is too hard to think about.

We have lost our connection to her memory, to the person within her. We were raised to believe there is a heaven and when you die, your body, however diseased or damaged in life, is restored whole again as you begin a new life. This new fresh life in heaven enriches and renews everything you did in this life a thousandfold through eternity.

And who will our mother be then? Will she be the mother of our childhood? Will she be the young, promising girl in high school she held onto as the disease crept through her past? Does death depend upon some sweet center of the brain to cast the life eternal? Will she remember everything but the last horrible years when she cursed us and said she had no children, or believed we had abandoned her or died?

In the meantime, there are moments, flickers of thought that grab you dead center and shake you hard with the realization your mother is sick and dying while you are driving down the street, eating dinner, going shopping, living normally. But, while you are going about your normal life, your mother is living in some kind of desperate no-memory-failing-bodily-function hell, and you're not doing anything about it. There's nothing you can do to give her back her life, or make a connection for her, that will tie her to the present— or the future. You cannot even go to her and sit with her and comfort her, and thereby comfort yourself, because she does not remember who you are anymore.

It is difficult to fully comprehend she does not, from moment to moment, remember anything that has happened or is happening. She cannot even remember she has eaten once she has swallowed.

You drive your car home. You call your sister. You send your mother a card you know she won't open. And you know, the deep way you feel those middle-of-the-night cold hard truths, that you have shamefully let go of any hope at all.

CHAPTER FIVE
AUGUST 1994

THERE ARE TWO NEW WOMEN ON WESLEY HALL. ONE looks so "normal" I see the kids do a double take because she doesn't wear a staff name tag. I know what they are thinking: What is she doing here?

Mom looked like her once. She even fooled the staff when they first met her in 1991. They thought we were wrong. They thought the doctors who had tested and examined her at the Turner Geriatric Clinic were wrong. Mom talked a good game. She was a great fake.

She was a brilliant woman. The summer after she graduated from high school in 1936 she took the Missouri State Teachers' exam and got the highest score on record. She was granted a teaching certificate that August and began teaching at a nearby school in Turtle Creek in September.

She was not only smart, she was tough. She was the boss and she ran everything under her jurisdiction or anything that got in her way. She raised four children by herself while our father was "on the road" for Leader Dogs, 300 out of 365 days a year. She cooked, cleaned, checked homework, fixed flat tires, flushed plumbing, gardened, volunteered, did Dad's expense account, balanced the checkbook, and managed music lessons, broken arms, and sibling rivalry without ever missing a beat or breaking down.

She was an amazing woman, and remained amazing up until the point where the Alzheimer's was so advanced even she couldn't get around it. We discovered, after we had finally been granted custody, our fears were right: she had been ill a long time. Her financial records for a good six or seven years back were a mess. She had always been a crackerjack bookkeeper. She had done all of our father's expense accounts and business records, and she took pride in balancing his expense account and our household budget to the penny.

When we went to the bank to review her accounts, we discovered she had been keeping a minimum of $30,000 in her checking account for the past few years. The bank officer who had always handled Mom's accounts told us she had tried unsuccessfully to get Mom to move her money to a money market where it would earn interest. Whenever she tried to talk to Mom about it, Mom would get angry and leave the bank. The bank officer said she thought it was crazy.

It wasn't crazy. It was smart. By keeping $30,000 in the bank, she could avoid the possibility she might bounce a check. She could eliminate all chance someone would accidentally discover she had forgotten how to add and subtract.

During this same period, from 1989 to 1991, she managed to rack up a wad of towing and car repair bills. When laid out on a table in chronological order, they were a suspicious lot. On a rather regular, sometimes weekly, basis Mom's car was towed because it wouldn't start. The starter was changed a couple times, as well as the battery, then later there were just towing charges and charges for "testing." In one five-month period, she had over $800 in repairs alone.

We believe she must have been having trouble with the sequence of actions it took to start the car: putting it in neutral, inserting the key, turning the key, pressing on the gas until the motor turned over, then putting the car in gear. In other words, she couldn't always remember how to start her car. And, the gas station was having a royal flush of a time collecting money for her confusion.

Put in the context of our mother being the sole driver for years, and having not only been the sole driver, but a driver who clocked in hundreds of thousands of miles taking our father from one speaking engagement to another, this little lapse of memory is staggering. The driver's seat was a second home for her.

The bills from the gas station anger me. The money in the bank, however, makes me sad, because it makes me think there was a time, a moment early in the disease, when she knew what was happening and was scrambling desperately to deny it, to stop it, in whatever way she could. And, the same fierce pride that made her boss made it impossible for her to tell anyone.

Difficulty with seemingly simple tasks which are really a sequence of tasks, like starting a car, is typical of Alzheimer's victims. An unwillingness or even refusal to bathe regularly is a dead giveaway something is seriously wrong.

71

In the fall of 1991, when we were coming to grips with our mother's illness while we were trying to gain custody of her, I was in Michigan to help my sister. It was a very difficult time and we were utterly exhausted with all the paperwork, the prognosis, and the staggering reality of what we were going to have to do to help her live comfortably.

Mom was living with Lolly at the time. I had just arrived and Lolly was clearly at her wit's end. She said she had been trying to talk Mom into taking a bath for the past week and had failed. She asked if I could oversee a bath for her so we could get her to change her clothes to go to the Turner Clinic at the University of Michigan for some testing.

I got towels, some fresh clothes, and took Mom into the bathroom. She was in a belligerent mood, which was typical of her during this time. When I urged her to come on and get into the shower, she began to get angry.

Mom was still big and strong and not one to tangle with either verbally or physically. Not wanting a fight, I just backed off a little and asked her to please take a shower so we could get dressed and go.

Luckily, her anger broke for a moment and I saw she was afraid. I waited until she could compose herself, then offered to help her take off her clothes.

She was amused. I helped her with her blouse and slacks, then had her sit down to take off her shoes and socks. Then she looked at me and said, pointing to her underwear and bra, "These too? I have to take off these?"

When I said yes, she asked why. When I told her they would get wet if she wore them into the shower, she was surprised, but agreed to take them off.

She didn't know what the soap was or what she was to do with it. She seemed afraid of the washcloth and didn't know what it was called or how it should be used. When I washed her hair, she became unhinged.

It was as though it was the first time she had ever bathed. It was all new and strange and confusing. When I wrapped her in a towel and got her out of the shower, she was close to tears. "It's very hard," she said. I understood: there were so many steps, so many tiny tasks making up bathing, it was hard to remember them all and to remember how and when to do them.

My mother has never acknowledged there is anything wrong with her. She has never talked about having Alzheimer's. In fact, during a visit with her in August of 1994, the staff at the Methodist Home said it was rather unnerving to them when Mom talked about her sister Geneva who has Alzheimer's. When she talks about Geneva, she cries, saying how terrible it is Geneva cannot remember anything, and how sad it is when someone has lost their past.

One day, during this same visit, we were sitting on a balcony in the sunshine with the children and she began crying uncontrollably. Then, just as suddenly, she stopped. When she stopped crying, she seemed surprised to look up and see the children were with us. She asked what their names were, and Lolly and I told her. She kept asking over and over, and we kept telling her, reminding her they were her grandchildren and three of them had family names from her family as their middle names.

It was clear this was confusing to her, so I asked her if she had a middle name. She thought about it for a minute and shook her head yes. I asked her what her middle name was, she hesitated for a minute then nodded her head before she spoke. "Laura," she said, "my middle name is Laura."

Lolly's real name is Laura. Mom's middle name is Margaret.

Although the doctors who examined her at the Turner Geriatric Clinic in 1991 described Mom as a "textbook" case, everyone reacts to Alzheimer's differently. Some get depressed and withdrawn, some angry and belligerent, some confused and weepy, and some just shut down. Also, there's no constant. Someone might be angry at first, then become weepy. Some are violent. Many of the people who have lived with Mom on Wesley Hall seem caved in. They wander. They sit. They mumble. They walk up and down the halls talking to themselves. They become obsessed with possessions and the biggest hassle seems to be what chairs "belong" to which people.

In the summer of 1994, Mom had taken possession of a large wooden rocking chair near the elevator. Earlier it was a different chair. One day a man made the mistake of sitting in "her" chair. When she saw him sit down, she flew down the hall and pushed him out of it.

We have witnessed any number of tussles regarding newspapers, shawls, books, chairs, and pocketbooks. The pocketbooks seem to be another "symptom" of the disease.

Mom carried one everywhere for the first couple of years. She had several of them, and if she came to visit Lolly and sat the purse down in order to eat or play with one of the children and "lost" it, she went into a panic.

The first year she lived at the Chelsea Methodist Home, we gave Mom twenty dollars in one-dollar bills so she would have money in her purse. The staff didn't like it because she was always giving it away to the other residents if they said they needed it. Many of the people we've met on Wesley Hall talk about money. More specifically, they talk about not having enough money. It is a source of worry and obsession.

We thought twenty dollars every couple months or so was a cheap price to pay for Mom's peace of mind. A wad of one-dollar bills stuffed in her purse seemed to give her the reassurance she had a lot of money. It also gave her a sense she could do something for someone else. She rather enjoyed giving her money away one dollar at a time, and we thought it was fine for her to do something that gave her pleasure.

Despite her toughness, she has always been very nurturing. She continues to be nurturing despite the ravages of her disease. The problems the staff has with her revolve around her concern for other patients and her desire to help them. Having people around her in distress, unfortunately, distresses her.

We have been very lucky Mom has been so nurturing, outgoing, and feisty during her decline. It's clear she isn't easy for the staff to handle. She's not easy for us to handle. But, she's interesting, and even when she can't make sense, her presence commands a certain amount of attention and respect, and the staff responds to her.

Whenever we leave Wesley Hall for a walk around the grounds everyone speaks to Mom. They all call her by her name, and she always responds, waves, and calls back with some little babble or banter. Sometimes her responses make sense, but often they don't.

The two new women, the ones who look normal, carry purses. They don't have them in hand, by the handles, but carry them in their arms close to their chests. They look worried when people pass them. They follow us around asking questions. They want to touch the children. The children are patient and stand still. They talk to them. The women smile. They start to talk. It doesn't make sense. It never does. The children are used to it, but I see Hedy is uncomfortable. I look at what she is looking at and I see the shorter woman, the one who is a little plump and carries a white purse, has written her name on her purse over and over again in ballpoint pen the same way Mom did a few years ago. I know what Hedy is thinking. I know she wonders if Mom can remember when she carried a purse. She also wonders how long this woman will carry her purse before she forgets it is hers. She wonders, like I do, how long it will all take.

Chapter Six
August 1994

Sarah, one of the women who has been on Wesley Hall as long as Mom has, is having a bad day. For the last couple of days we've visited, she's been in the halls searching for something. It has left her agitated and fragile.

Mom senses Sarah's agitation, and although she's in a relatively good frame of mind, she keeps watching her. We all watch Sarah, afraid she's going to blow.

The day before, Sarah tried to pull an electrical box off the wall with her hands. She said IT was hidden there. The attendant tried to soothe her as she deftly moved Sarah away from the box while another attendant pushed a tall upholstered chair in front of the box to keep it hidden from sight. Instead of solving the problem, hiding the box only heightened Sarah's search for IT.

Sarah's nervousness and obsessive searching make Mom jittery, so we take a walk down the hall. Sarah follows us, talking to herself, calling out to us as we cruise down to the end of the hall where the big picture window looks out onto a field.

Mom likes to look out the window and show me the trees, and tell me something about what's out there and about how the leaves sometimes "get" brown. Her sentences and ideas have jumbled like bits of broken glass and rarely follow a clean sequence, but manage in their context to make an idea or thought. I know when she talks about the trees being green sometimes and brown other times she knows fall is coming, although the words autumn, fall, winter, spring, and summer have long since left her brain.

Mom is just beginning to show me the trees when I hear Sarah behind us. I assume she's going to join us so I turn to say something to her. Just as I do, she turns away from me and runs to the fire escape door.

I'm frozen. I'm trapped between Mom and Sarah. I can't let go of Mom, who now uses my hand or my outstretched arm for balance, and I can't summon the nerve to grab Sarah and stop her. I don't know what Sarah would do. I have no idea if she would turn and hit me. She, like Mom, is unpredictable.

While I watch, Sarah hits the crash bar hard with both hands. The alarm screams out. Mom lets go of my arm and covers her ears. We are standing so close to the alarm, the ringing is terrifying as though the sound weren't coming from some small box, but from within us, warning us something bad is going to happen.

I see an attendant come running down the hall, fumbling with her keys. I look for Sarah. She is standing there, her hands still on the bar, a smile spreading across her face. She is enjoying the ringing of the alarm the way I might enjoy a symphony.

Mom starts to cry. The attendant puts one arm around Sarah, steps between Sarah and the door, and reaches up to the alarm with her other hand to shut it off with a key.

I don't know what to do besides tell the attendant I'm sorry, I couldn't stop her. She assures me it's fine, because the patients never go through the door. The sound of the alarm stops them.

I can see her looking down the hall at the other, resident she left in order to stop the alarm. I tell her I'll take Sarah for her. Mom and I will walk a little with her. The attendant thanks me and heads back down the hall.

Sarah is still searching for IT. I take Mom's hand and tell her everything is fine. As the three of us head down the hall, Sarah kisses her fingertips and touches the fire door affectionately. She seems calmer, which serves to reassure Mom that all is fine again.

As we amble down the hall, I tell Sarah I'll help her look in her room for IT. I'm sure, I try to reassure her, IT is in her room.

I have never been in Sarah's room. There's no reason for me to have ever been there and I am unprepared for what I see.

As I turn the knob and swing the door open, I am confronted with a room filled with oil paintings: beautiful, powerful oil paintings. And I know, before I summon the nerve to look at the bold signature scrawled across the bottom, they are Sarah's.

There are landscapes, a still life or two, all of them far more than competent. They are exquisite. They are the work of a gifted artist.

The painting that stays with me, the one I see when I close my eyes now, is one of the largest ones, hung on the wall opposite her door. It is a picture of a dark-skinned man, perhaps a Mexican, with a bandana tied across his forehead. He is leaning back. His face is serene, and in his hands he holds the reins of two white horses, their faces distorted with strain trying to push forward as he calmly holds them back.

Sarah pushes me aside to look into her room. IT isn't there, she tells me, then moves on down the hall, still searching.

An attendant comes toward me. I am still standing in Sarah's doorway, my mother is holding my hand.

"They're hers, aren't they," I say to the attendant.

She nods yes, then turns her head away, as though she too cannot face the loss of the life of this artist.

We both know she is gone. The woman, strong, brilliant, talented, who painted these pictures is dead.

In the same way, the woman who was boss, who ran our family, ran our lives, ran everything, who is now groping for words to describe the strange phenomenon of falling leaves, of seasons and the passing of time, is gone.

Sarah's pictures are chilling. Sarah's pictures are a tangible expression of the grief we feel when we visit Mom. Sarah's pictures are like the AIDS quilt that now covers nearly a mile of loss, fifteen feet wide. Its weight could smother you.

When I think about Sarah's pictures, I think about the empty words of my doctor trying to reassure me I will not be a victim of Alzheimer's. "People who have active mental lives, people who continue to work and are creative," she says, citing the studies, "are less likely to have Alzheimer's than those who do not." The argument sounds reasonable. It sounds like it might have some medical basis, some credible rationale. It sounds like something I can comfortably cling to.

It isn't true. Sarah's pictures prove it. And the loss you feel when you look at the pictures and see

Sarah wandering the halls looking for IT is a loss so deep, so wide it could swallow you whole.

I take my mother's hand and walk her down the hall. I do not want her to see these pictures. I do not want her to know the woman who just crashed through the fire escape door was once an artist. I do not want her to know she herself was once a brilliant woman who ran a household and worked in her community and was respected by everyone who knew her. I do not want her to know what is happening to her. I want to sit by her, hold her hand, tell her everything is going to be fine, and hope she believes me.

CHAPTER SEVEN
AUGUST 1994

MEDICINE IS A SCIENCE. AND, LIKE ALL GOOD SCIENCES, it carefully develops its own nomenclature, a means of classification. Medical science likes careful guidelines to help the physicians make correct diagnoses. With most diseases, the physician sees a patient during the early stages and is knowledgeable of those stages and how they progress. These early signs help the physician make an early diagnosis and take proper medical precautions. Sometimes diagnosis in an early stage can forestall or even stop the spread of a disease and improve the chances of recovery and survival.

In this early diagnosis and prevention model, Alzheimer's presents some unique problems. First, patients and patients' families rarely seek medical help during the "early onset" stages, and furthermore, even if they did, there is not, to date, anything the physician can do to stop or even slow down the debilitating dementia parade.

In August 1994, after Mom had been a resident of the Alzheimer's wing since 1991, Lolly and I met with the head nurse and resident director to talk about Mom. Mom had been extremely depressed that summer. She cried all the time and was agitated. They had tried various medications on her with little success. We asked to meet with them because we were worried they might at some time, out of exasperation, resort to restraining her in order to control her. We did not want them to do so. We believed she was claustrophobic and any attempt to restrain her would only serve to make her lash out in anger. The thought of them having to restrain her made my stomach knot and twist.

The staff sensed our discomfort. The director looked at the chart spread out on her lap then up at us. She said they were having as hard a time with Mom's decline as we were because it all seemed so rapid, so sudden, especially since she had only had Alzheimer's for three years.

Her remark was like a whiplash. Three years! I felt a scream strangling in my throat. I felt betrayed. I could see my sister move to the edge of her seat before she spoke. I knew her voice was going to be high and loud and strained.

It had not been three years. It had been more like ten. But, both Lolly and I knew before we started to talk, as far as they were concerned, it had been three years.

Medical professionals have a different take on this disease than those who live it. For them, the disease begins when the patient and/or the family comes to them for help. The office visit in which the physician confirms the family's suspicions signals the starting point. In their defense, there's no way for them to know any better because they have not lived through the circumstances that brought the family to see them.

For the families, it is different. There are months and oftentimes years of fuzzy moments. Moments when they are not quite sure they heard it right or felt it right or that things were ever right.

Then, there's denial. Not on the part of the victim, but of the victim's family. Hardcore denial. The kind only a good psychiatrist could enjoy confronting.

It is not always easy to understand what is happening. Alzheimer's does not come on full blown, nor does it attack in a clean clear-cut manner. It is often muddied by a family's history. It is camouflaged by the quirks of aging and all those rough edges you don't want, or just plain refuse, to see in someone you love.

And, unless you're living with the afflicted person day to day, it's difficult to gather enough "evidence" to support your growing concerns. Unfortunately, once you feel certain what you are experiencing and seeing is dementia, it is not immediately clear what action you should take.

With our mother we saw a gradual edginess turn into a sharp sword of anger. We learned not to question her confusion, memory lapses, or losses unless we wanted to be hit broadside with that sword. Out of self-protection, we did not make ourselves fully aware of how confused she was in those early onset years.

Unfortunately, it is easiest to identify the early onset years once you've passed them. Hindsight, however, is not helpful. What do those early onset years look like? What types of behavior signal something is going wrong?

As outlined by the Alzheimer's Association, the ten warning signs of Alzheimer's are:

1. Recent memory loss that affects job skills. They note that it is normal to occasionally forget names, phone numbers, assignments, or appointments, but that dementia, such as Alzheimer's, causes people to forget things more often and not remember them later. Alzheimer's victims might also ask the same question repeatedly, not remembering the answer or realizing they have asked the question before.

2. Difficulty performing familiar tasks.

3. Problems with language, i.e., forgetting simple words or substituting inappropriate words, thereby making a sentence incomprehensible.

4. Disorientation of time and place. For example, getting lost in a familiar shopping mall or while taking a walk in the neighborhood or other familiar place.

5. Poor or decreased judgment.

6. Problems with abstract thinking.

7. Misplacing things. They duly note a person with Alzheimer's disease may do more than misplace something. They might put things in inappropriate places such as putting an iron in the freezer or a wristwatch in the sugar bowl.

8. Changes in mood or behavior: rapid unexplained mood swings from calm to tears, anger to calm, and back again in a few moments.

9. Changes in personality.

10. Loss of initiative.

This ten-warning-signs model comes from the American Cancer Society's "Ten Warning Signs Of Cancer" public awareness program. But, changes in mood, behavior, or personality are considerably harder to monitor than the growth of a mole. Many of the Alzheimer's symptoms can be easily overlooked, or worse, misdiagnosed as symptoms of depression.

The American Psychiatric Association (APA), in its publication on Alzheimer's, gives a list of symptoms of depression capable of mimicking or complicating Alzheimer's disease which includes:

* Unexplained weakness or fatigue, dizzy spells, low energy

* Stomachaches, indigestion, constipation; urinary disturbances

* Change in eating habits, appetite, and weight

* Sleep disturbances

* Slowed or more agitated movement

* Feelings of tension, anxiety, or irritability

* Loss of initiative, inability to enjoy activities once enjoyed

* Indecisiveness, apathy, boredom, indifference

* Poor attention and concentration

* Tendency to cry and become upset over minor issues and events; low self-esteem; feelings of worthlessness, hopelessness, helplessness, inappropriate guilt

* Thoughts of suicide

The APA checklist of Alzheimer's disease symptoms describes:

* Loss of short-term memory occurs; person can't learn new information

* Loss of long-term memory occurs; person can't remember personal information such as birth place or occupation

* Judgment is impaired

* Aphasia develops: patient can't recall words or understand the meaning of common words

* Apraxia develops: patient loses control over muscles and can't, for example, button shirts or operate zippers

* Patients lose spatial abilities and can't assemble blocks, arrange sticks in a certain order or copy a three-dimensional figure

* Personality changes: patient may become un- usually angry, irritable, quiet, confused

The American Psychiatric Association ends its list with a disclaimer: "Presence of any or all of these symp- toms is not a sure indicator of Alzheimer's disease; only a complete examination by a psychiatrist or other physician can confirm the diagnosis."

Both associations provide helpful insights into the early stages, but Alzheimer's defies easy diagnosis. In fact, despite numerous new medical and cognitive di- agnostic tests, the only definitive "test" for Alzheimer's is still an autopsy.

In light of the aging "process," many of the warn- ing signs seem part of the normal baggage of growing old: forgetfulness; an occasional fumbling with a but- ton or zipper; change in eating and sleeping habits; misplacing car keys, a purse, the grocery list. And, it is natural for family members to see some of these behaviors as just affectations of aging instead of blink- ing red lights of trouble.

Even if you suspect something is wrong and you can clearly identify your family member has exhibited one or more of the characteristic behaviors of Alzheimer's, what do you do? Imagine how difficult it would be to convince a parent or a spouse they need to go to a doctor because you suspect their recent oversight of your birthday/anniversary or memory lapse over how to light a pilot light on their stove means they have dementia.

I have yet to meet anyone who claims to have made an "early diagnosis" of Alzheimer's in a family member. Instead, I know dozens of people who sadly admit they can piece together the decline once they "looked back" over what might have been years of irrational behavior. If you're living it, the best insight, unfortunately, is hindsight.

In retrospect, the pieces of the puzzle fit: the sudden explosion of anger; the forgotten appointment; the misplaced keys/glasses/purse/shoes; the jumbling of past and present; the loss of interest in everyday activities such as cooking, sewing, gardening, visiting with friends; the repeated questions.

In retrospect, we should have known something was wrong when our mother didn't want to bring out her Christmas tree in 1989. Mom loved Christmas. She especially loved her tree. And, she was a bit eccentric about it.

Years ago she bought a good artificial tree and spent hours carefully decorating it with all the ornaments we had made in school, as well as the ones she had bought and collected, tying them on with red velvet ribbons. She thought the tree was so beautiful she never took it down, but kept it instead, all year-round, covered with a sheet in the corner of the basement, which was more of a family room than a basement. It was the place Mom and Ray entertained.

When you're starting with someone who's eccentric, it's hard to tell when they cross the line. My mother's penchant for doing what she felt like and saying what she thought made it just that much more difficult for us to be sure her behavior was out of her range of normal.

But, in 1989, she just didn't want to bother getting the tree out of the corner, or putting any decorations around the house. She also told me I was stupid for wanting to because it was too much work, too much fuss, too much silliness. This wasn't like her at all, but there was so much that wasn't like her during that time, it was hard to sort out what was happening.

We let the incident pass. We decided she was just being crotchety. Her behavior wasn't life threatening, and certainly nothing to give you cause to drag her to the doctor. In retrospect, it was one of those early signs we missed. Or, one that we ignored.

If I knew then what I know now, how not bringing out the Christmas tree probably meant she also didn't know how to light her stove if the pilot light went out, or take a bath, I would have done something. But I didn't know, and, even armed with the sharpest of hindsight, I do not have a better list than either the Alzheimer's Association's or the American Psychiatric Association's for determining if someone you love is in trouble. I do not have any answers or hard-core truths.

The "onset" of Alzheimer's is a tricky one. If you suspect something is wrong, you should see a physician immediately. Make a list of the "strange" activities and uncharacteristic episodes that concern you. Give the doctors as much information as possible. They will have no magic medicine to change what is happening, but they will be able to eliminate other possible causes. And, they can alert you to other things to watch for. Even though you cannot stop

Alzheimer's, understanding what is happening can help you take better care of the person you love who is ill.

It is, however, as I also know, difficult to convince someone they ought to see a doctor because their memory is playing tricks on them. It's also sometimes difficult to convince a doctor this experience of memory loss is more than the normal aging process. The early undiagnosed years of our mother's disease were frustrating and confusing. Until there was a major crisis, we didn't have access to our mother's doctor. We were neither able to get her there with one of us in attendance, nor were we able to find out from the doctor, once Mom did see him for a checkup, what he thought. Caught in this strange bind, we often thought we saw signs of terrible trouble, but because we were powerless to do anything about it, we looked away.

So, when we had a chance to speak with the director of the Alzheimer's wing, and she voiced her surprise at Mom's rapid decline, we told our story once again. Hoping she and the staff would make notes and understand Mom had not had Alzheimer's for three years, but for ten.

More than likely all the families with patients on her ward have experiences similar to ours. Victims of Alzheimer's, which includes the patients and their families, need to begin talking to the medical professionals. We need to tell our stories so the knowledge base increases and we are all more aware of what is happening, when it is happening—not afterward, when it is too late to do anything to help.

Chapter Eight

November 1994

I HAVE DREAMS SOMETIMES WHERE MOM IS SICK, BUT she's sick in a wheelchair, or maybe has cancer, or her arm is bandaged, but her face is full and animated. In these dreams, we laugh together and talk.

We have long conversations, sit close to one another and hold hands. We talk about taking a trip. She tells me, like she used to tell me when I was a child, how she would like to see the windmills in Holland. I tell her I'll take her and we begin to make plans.

When I wake from these dreams, my stomach hurts. I will never take my mother to see the windmills. Not only that, but I am afraid to take her out of the Methodist Home. I am afraid she might hit someone or grab the steering wheel of the car while I am driving. I am afraid she might panic, get angry, lash out, and cry uncontrollably because it's getting dark and she wants to go home, but she doesn't recognize the building where she lives.

She used to know my daughter's name. Hedy is her only granddaughter, and Mom would once beam with recognition when she saw her. When she couldn't recognize me as her daughter, she could still name Hedy.

In return, Hedy loves her unconditionally. Ironically, in 1984, when I was pregnant with Hedy, my mother came to visit. It was the last time she ever came to our home.

By then she had three grandsons. She had always wanted a granddaughter and kept telling me when I was pregnant it had to be a girl for her. I had a rough pregnancy. I was exhausted and sick. I had a blood clot in one leg and spent the majority of the pregnancy in bed. Before Mom's visit, I made the mistake of telling her I honestly didn't care whether it was a boy or a girl, I just wanted it to come.

Since I was unable to travel because of the complications with the pregnancy, my mother and Ray came to North Carolina to visit us. They were doing some extensive construction in the airport at the time which caused a rerouting of arriving passengers, and kept me from meeting Mom and my stepfather, Ray, at the gate. Instead, I had to stand at the end of a long construction ramp to pick them up. As soon as she stepped off the plane and onto the ramp, my mother started yelling at me. You could hear her all over the airport.

"If it's not a girl," she screamed, "it's because you haven't wished it to be a girl. I know you, you're doing this to hurt me. You haven't wished, have you?

You just want to hurt me. You just want to make sure I don't ever have a granddaughter. That's just like you." I was very pregnant and it was obvious I was the focus of her attention. People started to laugh. When she heard them laugh, she got madder. By the time she got to the end of the ramp and I tried to hug her hello, she was steaming. She pushed me aside and told me not to bother.

She stayed mad at me during the entire visit. In fact, she remained mad at me for the next couple of years. It was an unexplained anger with no focus. My brothers and sister kept saying I must have done something to make her angry. I didn't understand what was happening and I couldn't imagine, for the life of me, what I had done.

Her actions at the airport and during her visit were not only irrational, they were unlike her. She had always been opinionated, and sometimes critical, but never mean-spirited. In fact, despite her gruffness, she was always loving. I began to worry something might be wrong with her, but it would be years before we knew for sure: years, and many, many harsh and hurtful words later.

Despite my mother's belief that I was not wishing hard enough, I had a girl, and Mom loved her. And, Hedy, despite the fact she never knew her grandmother when she was well, loved her back.

Then, when we came to visit her in the fall of 1994, Mom didn't know Hedy. It was hard to watch. I didn't know what to do. I needed to be there for my mother even though she didn't know who I was, yet I had to protect my daughter.

Caught in the cross fire, I had to watch as my mother sputtered and cried and mumbled and jumbled her way through a myriad of thoughts and confusion. My nine-year-old daughter, heartbroken her grandmother didn't know who she was, moved further and further away until she was, during one scary, volatile moment, standing in a corner of my mother's room with her hands covering her face as if to protect herself from what she heard and saw.

I worry about my children's memories of their grandmother. Mom, since the Alzheimer's, is sometimes sweet, childlike, and calm. She is also erratic, angry, irrational, and crazy in her speech and actions. Much of the time she is so tense and wound up she feels dangerous.

I was much older than Hedy when my grandmother, my mother's mother, started showing signs of dementia. Unlike Hedy, I was one of many granddaughters. My grandmother had fourteen children, and all fourteen children bore children. By the time I was ten or eleven I was one of a throng of grandchildren.

The memories of my grandmother that I struggle to hold onto smell like baking powder biscuits and buttermilk. We visited her each summer at her home in Big Creek, and when we arrived, grandmother would come out onto the sagging wooden porch of her tiny house and dry her hands on her apron before adjusting her delicate gold-framed glasses.

"Let me see," she'd say, her voice quivering, lips working a little nervously. "Come here," she'd call, holding out her arms so I could bury myself in the flour-dusted folds of her apron. "You're the tallest one, you must be Carrie Jane, Ruth's daughter. Yes, Carrie Jane."

When Grandfather died the fall of 1966, Grandma "lost her mind." When Grandma became ill, my mother's thirteen brothers and sisters and their spouses, who were scattered all over the United States, pulled in their resources to help care for her.

Grandma lived in Big Creek in the Ozarks near Bunker, Missouri. She and Grandpa settled there ten years after they got married and stayed. Other than the little traveling they did, following Grandpa's jobs with the railroad the first ten years of their marriage, Grandma had never been anywhere on a bus, train, or plane. In fact, except for an occasional ride to church or town in Grandpa's car, I don't think she ever left the Bunker area again until Grandpa died.

When Grandpa died, Grandma's world fell apart. She starting crying all the time, saying she wanted to go see John in Connecticut, or Polly in Minnesota, or my mother, Ruth, in Michigan. On Mom's urging, the family put Grandma on a plane and sent her to stay with us.

It was the one and only time Grandma ever flew. I was fifteen years old when Grandma came to visit. My mother went to the airport to pick her up. She was very excited at the prospect of having her mother stay with us. It was the only time her mother had ever visited her home and she was anxious to show it off to her.

Unfortunately, by the time they got from the airport to our house, Grandma had already begun insisting she wanted to go somewhere else. Mom was struggling to remain calm when she unpacked Grandma's bags, but began to become unraveled when Grandma started insisting she didn't know my mother. When Mom said she was her daughter, Grandma looked at her incredulously and said quite clearly that she had no living children. They were all dead.

At this pronouncement, Mom began to get edgy. She kept telling Grandma over and over again that she was her daughter. As further proof of this fact, she would patiently go down the list of children, all living, and tell their names and their spouses' names and all their living children's names.

Grandma just stared at her. Later, she told Mom they had gone to high school together. When Mom corrected her, saying she was her daughter, not someone she grew up with, Grandma got angry and nervous.

It was a terrifying time. Grandma was like a frightened animal. Whenever my father would walk into the room, she would scream, grab my arm and ask who he was, or who my mother was, or beg me to take her to Polly's house. Time and space meant nothing to her. She was afraid to eat. She told me once she thought "they" were trying to poison her. She wandered the house at night coming into our rooms and waking us, crying and begging us to take her home.

In less than a week's time, Grandma was on a plane back to Missouri. This was the last time I saw my grandmother, and whenever the memories of her, frightened, confused, and lost, crowd into my mind, I try to force them out. I bury my face again in the memory of her big dusty apron. I want more than anything to believe, although she did not always know my name, my grandmother loved me.

She died a couple of years later in the Madison Memorial Hospital. The ghost of her fear and confusion filled our house and our lives for a long time after.

I do not believe we should raise children to expect "happily ever after" throughout their lives. Witnessing this kind of mental unraveling, however, is the grand stuff of nightmares, which leaves you wondering what to tell your children.

When one of Mom's doctors suggested we tell our children that Grandma's brain was like a malfunctioning tape recorder erasing what you say, then erasing a couple of days in the past each time she sleeps, I thought it an easy image and concept to grasp. It is an acceptable way to think about Grandma's crazy statements, her nervousness, her inability to remember we visited her yesterday, or just ate dinner, or that I am her daughter and they are her grandchildren.

As she deteriorates, unfortunately, the children's questions get more complicated and harder to explain. They want to know how Grandma is going to die. They want to know what it will be like when they visit her the next time. They want to know if we can still take her out for an ice cream or to Lolly's house for Christmas morning.

They are jumpy when the phone rings at odd times. My daughter wants to know if I'll get Alzheimer's, and if I do, what should she do. My youngest son makes me promise I won't get sick, ever. They want to know if Alzheimer's is contagious, if they can get it.

I tell them no, I hope I won't get Alzheimer's. I promise them I'll take good care of myself, but tell them I can't promise I won't ever get sick. And, I tell them over and over again that Alzheimer's is not contagious and that it is fine for them to hug their grandmother.

Since Grandma clearly had some form of dementia and Mom and two of her sisters are victims of Alzheimer's, I worry we might be in line for trouble. The threat of Alzheimer's seems far away for now. My children's dreams and memories are more pressing.

My mother's illness has taken an enormous toll on our lives. I can see it in my face: it has aged me...not very gracefully. I sense it in my younger brother's nervousness, his discomfort in having to visit Mom at the home. I hear it in my sister's tired voice on the telephone. The toll for her has been the greatest. Since the fall of 1991, when Mom came to live with her then later went to the Methodist Home, Lolly has suffered with high blood pressure and lower back pain.

I understand it clearly when my older brother, Gary, shakes his head and says again, "She was always the boss." It has aged and saddened us all.

It has also robbed our children of a grandmother. The loss of her "life" has been a loss so deep and strong, I wonder sometimes if we will have the strength when it is all over to pull back the good memories and tell the stories of when she was wild and well and someone who loved us all.

CHAPTER NINE

SEPTEMBER 1994

I SAW MOM FOUR WEEKS AGO. LOLLY HAS CALLED ME or I have called her at least twice a week since then to keep up with what's happening.

Mom has started falling. When Lolly went to visit her, a couple of days after I left, she noticed Mom's right foot would flop in an odd fashion whenever she sat down and crossed her legs. Lolly thinks Mom also seemed extremely pigeon toed and awkward in her gait. She thinks this might be the cause of Mom's falls.

The staff asked Lolly to take Mom to an orthopedist for an evaluation. By the time of the appointment, Mom had fallen several more times, and the staff was trying to get her to use a walker.

Mom angrily rejected the walker. They tried a wheelchair, which didn't anger her, although she kept trying to get out of it and falling. In order to encourage her to stay in the wheelchair, the staff added a "soft" restraint meant to remind Mom to stay seated in her chair. The restraint agitated her.

We have always known Mom is claustrophobic. She is one of those people who can't stand tight clothes or tight places. She nearly ripped the seat belts out of the car when they were first introduced.

We have all dreaded the day when she would either become immobile or immobilized. Everyone has their own version of Orwell's "Room 101." Being constrained, immobile, without will or "wheels" was Mom's. To see it coming, to know it's going to happen, and realize you are going to have to watch it happen, is staggering.

Lolly called to tell me the staff had obtained permission from her attending physician to restrain Mom. Her behavior had become so erratic, the staff felt they could no longer control her. They also couldn't keep her in her chair. They were afraid she would fall and break a hip, shoulder, or arm, or even take someone else down with her. This new twist in her battle with Alzheimer's was one we knew was inevitable, but nonetheless one we had trouble accepting.

A few days after the restraining order, when Lolly put Mom in the car to go to see an orthopedist and tried to buckle her seat belt for her, Mom freaked. She thought Lolly was trying to restrain her or tie her into the car and she fought against her. "Buckling up" was quite a battle. Lolly was rattled and exhausted before she ever left the parking lot.

The orthopedist, unfortunately, did not have particularly good news. A surgically fused ruptured disk, done thirty years earlier, was probably the source of the problem with her foot. Since Mom was unable to answer any questions during the examination, the doctor guessed the nerve allowing Mom to flex her foot and point her toe had given out. Who knows if it was in any way connected with neurological damage from the Alzheimer's. It was, however, made far more complicated by the Alzheimer's.

The solution to the problem seemed simple enough: Mom was to wear a brace. If the brace didn't make mobility possible, she would then have to use a walker or a wheel chair. Easier said than done.

Lolly talked to Mom about the problem. She tried to explain that her foot had quit working and if she kept trying to walk she would fall. Lolly was calm and repeated the information over and over, stressing how important it was for Mom not to try to walk, because, if she tried to walk unaided, she would fall.

The more Lolly talked to Mom about the importance of not trying to walk, the more agitated Mom became. Eventually she responded by declaring she was strong. And she is strong. Strong as an ox and stubborn as a knot in a pine tree.

When Lolly brought Mom back to the Methodist Home after her visit to the orthopedist, the staff informed Lolly they were not sure they could continue to keep Mom on the Alzheimer's wing. The falling incidents, her heightened agitation and irrational behavior, punctuated on occasion by physical outbursts, and her unwillingness to stay in the wheelchair, made it impossible for them to take good care of her.

When Lolly asked about other options, they suggested she could/should be moved to the nursing-care wing where the staff was larger and better equipped to deal with Mom. Unfortunately, there were, they told Lolly, no vacancies right then, so Mom might have to be moved to a nursing home away from the Chelsea Methodist Home until a spot was available for her.

Ray, our stepfather, had been in a nursing home. It was smelly, ugly, and the "care" was questionable. Lolly worked hard to get him out of the nursing home once she was his legal guardian, but she didn't succeed before he died. She was not anxious to have Mom anywhere but the Chelsea Methodist Home. She also knew they couldn't move her to another facility without heavily sedating her, which wouldn't be good either. She pushed for other options.

The staff said they might be able to keep Mom on the Alzheimer's wing until a spot in nursing became available if we were able to provide twenty-four-hour private nursing care for her. The cost: $260 a day.

Lolly and I went back and forth on the telephone trying to figure out what to do. Mom only had about $80,000 left in disposable income: the rest was tied up in her house. We quickly realized at $260 a day, $80,000 would only cover 307 days of care: less than a year. Buying private nursing care didn't seem like a viable option.

We were in a Catch-22. We had always said we would sell her house to pay for her care, but renting her house did a better job of providing her an income to pay for her care...as long as her care remained around $35,000 a year. The rent from her house, Ray's pension, and a small pension Mom got from our father, along with her social security check, were, until now, covering most of her expenses. We were prepared to sell her house, but selling the house had some strings attached.

Mom's house was in a community with buyer protection laws where all houses must pass stringent building inspections before they can be sold. All repairs, under this buyer protection system, are the responsibility of the seller.

We had already had the house inspected and knew it needed a new roof, some masonry work, and some updating on wiring and plumbing. Also, fifteen years earlier, there had been slight water damage in the basement along one wall. Although there was no additional damage or active deterioration, in order to get a certificate to sell, we would have to have the foundation excavated on the back of the house, have the exterior foundation wall waterproofed and repairs done, and we would have to have a new drainage system dug.

Mom had not kept the house up during her last few years of living in it, but we were shocked at what we would have to do in order to sell it. So, slowly, over the years of renting it, we had one repair done after another in preparation for the time we would have to sell it. We had replaced the roof, put in air conditioning, had the masonry work done, painted the garage, but had not done the foundation repairs.

Home repairs are not only costly, they're time consuming. You can schedule a repairman to come, but he comes when he wants to come, which may be six hours, six weeks, or even six months from the time you wanted him there. Consequently, Mom's house was far from easily accessed disposable income.

Lolly was prepared to try negotiating with the staff in the hopes of keeping Mom in the Alzheimer's wing until something became available in nursing. If we could hire a private nurse for the "worst times" of the day rather than around the clock, we might be able to buy Mom a little more time. The last thing we wanted to do was move her twice. A move of any kind would be difficult, but two moves would be a disaster.

Lolly didn't even have a chance to discuss this option. By the next day, Mom had become extremely agitated at the staff's attempts to confine her to a wheelchair and she kicked and punched several people. In the midst of our nursing-care, what-to-do-with-Mom-now crisis, someone on the nursing floor in the Methodist Home died. Mom was immediately bumped to the top of the "priority list" for this placement and was moved two days later to the medical wing.

It was a tragic way for us to find a solution to our problem. But like so many things with Alzheimer's, all solutions have their strings, downsides, and compromises.

In the wake of these tumultuous two days, I considered dropping everything and going to Michigan. Lolly kept saying no, it was under control. Besides, she insisted, there would be worse problems to handle in the future. With Alzheimer's, just when you think you have the situation in hand and you're on smooth ground, providing the best care you can, something new crops up and you're back to square one.

During this period of difficulty with her foot and the subsequent falls, Mom became more agitated and more weepy. Through this and other changes, my respect for the staff and the "institution" of the Chelsea Methodist Home continues to grow. Through all their difficulties with Mom, they have never once resorted to "snowing" her, the term the nursing staff uses to describe sedating a patient to the point of immobilizing them. Also, the restraints they use on her are minimal.

This does not make the situation easier. We are still left wondering what Mom thinks. We have quit asking her because she cannot tell us. The most frustrating moment in it all came when Lolly tried to tell Mom not to try walking because her foot wouldn't work, not to get out of the chair because she would fall down, and to please stay in the wheelchair so she could remain where she was for awhile longer. Mom's response to Lolly's pleading was to stand up and try to walk to show Lolly how strong she was. And again, with Lolly watching, she fell. She fell because she didn't understand. Lolly couldn't make her understand. Tragically, whatever last moment there was when she did or could understand is gone. There will be no glorious remission of reasoning. There are no beautiful "Disney" moments with Alzheimer's. No pretty closing scenes or easy solutions. It is impractical and probably inhumane to attempt to keep someone like Mom in our homes. We would have to restrain her at night to keep her from wandering, from falling down the stairs, from walking out the door and getting lost. Also, we have no means to contain or control her outbursts, and no way to protect our children from her dangerous hurting words, or the occasional blows of her raging fists.

It does not, however, keep us from wondering if we can do better than we are doing now, fighting to keep her in a place we know is clean, safe, and equipped at all hours of the day and night to both restrain and help her.

The Methodist Home is, undeniably, a form of "restraint." It might be a "soft" restraint, but it is, nonetheless, a restraint. The home confines her movements. It controls her environment. It keeps her from moving freely in the world.

When she lived on the Alzheimer's wing, the elevator was locked so she couldn't leave. On the medical wing, she wears an alarm system clipped to the back of her wheelchair. It goes off if she leaves the ward, signaling to the nurses that she's escaped.

For the most part, she is unaware of these restraints. They no longer use the soft restraint, a cloth-covered foam pad wedged in between the front arms of her wheelchair forming a soft table/restraint, which made it difficult for her to get out of her chair. They now use a seat belt on her wheelchair to keep her contained. She rarely tries to stand because she has lost her sense of balance. Even without her flopping foot, she could not keep herself upright for long.

We are both comfortable and uncomfortable with these restraining devises. We are aware of their necessity, but wonder what the lives of the patients would be like without them. We try to imagine an institution designed to accommodate their night wanderings, their daytime obsessions with pacing and searching. We dream about "playgrounds" for Alzheimer's victims where they can roam and explore and release some of their anger and energy without hurting themselves or others.

At present, what is available for Alzheimer's victims is a "medical" model consistent with old age and geriatric needs. This model is filled with wheelchairs, feeding tubes, adult diapers, bedpans, and medication. It is in many ways an appropriate and decent model. But, maybe there's a better one.

We know, if we had Mom in one of our homes, we would have to use many more forms of restraint to keep her from hurting herself, from hurting us, and from damaging our collective environment. Because, unfortunately, in her loss of understanding, Mom can be destructive to herself, others, and her environment.

One difference we have observed between the Alzheimer's patients and the other geriatric patients on the medical wing is that the Alzheimer's patients are more restless. They scoot their wheelchairs incessantly from one end of the hall to the other. They also propel their walkers and walking devices at an alarming and erratic speed. They are, for the most part, more aggressive than the other patients.

Maybe they need a couple hours every day on an indoor track racing each other in their various devices to work off their aggression and agitation. Maybe they need wider halls and bigger spaces to roam. Maybe they need gardens to dig, little inclines to maneuver, windows to open and close, or environmental changes and challenges. Maybe, as their minds wind backwards, furiously erasing their memories, their brain motors are racing forward and need some release.

Maybe there are other ways to help Alzheimer's victims spend their last frustrating days rather than modifying existing hospital environments so we might keep these patients more contained.

CHAPTER TEN

OCTOBER 13, 1994

IT IS LOLLY'S BIRTHDAY. MOM'S BIRTHDAY IS OCTOBER 17 and I dread it. When I saw her in August, she kept asking if it was her birthday. She kept insisting it was her birthday. My sleep has been flooded with nightmares of her birthday, her death. In my dreams they are the same. It feels like a car wreck, like my rib cage has been jerked too hard, the wind knocked out of me, and I am crying without being able to breathe.

My mother used to say she was a little psychic. It is the only trait I got from her. I do not have her black hair, broad cheekbones, or hazel eyes. I have instead an uneasy ability to feel the future: a twisted gift to sense what is happening before it happens. But knowing she is going to die takes no gift.

We are beginning to see the first signs of her physical decline. She is a little herky-jerky when she tries to move or hold things. She can't walk without assistance. Her speech pattern has also changed, signaling some new damage in her brain. She gets stuck on sounds, stuttering them out in an odd cadence, "Do-do-do-do yo-yo-you want to-to-to-to go."

She, like all of us, will die. It is difficult, however, despite the rampant destruction of her brain, to predict when or how she will die. The nagging suspicion hers will not be a swift and merciful death, however, is our greatest concern. As each new manifestation of her decline comes forward, we are even more aware of how uncomfortable her life with this disease must be. Each new "symptom" is greeted with a rising agitation from her, making her more and more difficult to handle and hold.

When I was shopping with my friend, Ingrid, one Saturday morning, we stumbled on an artist's yard sale. The artist's front porch was full of handmade baskets, quilts, and dolls she had made and wanted to be rid of. She hoped to pare down her life a little and make it more manageable. My mother used to love dolls. This woman's dolls were soft and touchable. I was having a hard time looking at them, thinking about how, if my mother were well, if she were herself, she would love being on this woman's lawn, touching her dolls, taking time to make the best selection, find the prettiest one to buy and take home.

That's when I found the teddy bear. It was on the ground surrounded by dolls and miniature baskets. It was a patchwork teddy bear, with a barrel of a tummy, and it was soft, so soft you could sense the years of loving in it. It was made from an old blue-and-white quilt touched and washed so many times it was nearly threadbare.

I bought it, brought it home, changed its startled blue button eyes to soft brown ones, and tied one blue and one white satin ribbon around its neck, wrapped it in tissue, and sent it to my sister to give to my mother. I hoped if Lolly took it to her, Mom might understand it was a present: hers to keep and hold and talk to.

Mom would get candy, flowers, and a teddy bear for her birthday. Ironically, Lolly would spend her own birthday meeting with the Chelsea Methodist Home's medical staff to discuss Mom's condition. Every ninety days Lolly has to meet with the staff to review Mom's "case."

The nursing wing is a medical wing, and when they moved her from the Alzheimer's unit to the medical wing, they did a complete workup on Mom. These medical tests revealed Mom had, in addition to Alzheimer's, extreme hardening of the arteries in the brain, high blood pressure, and emphysema from years of smoking.

There was some speculation regarding her inability to walk, and some suspicion this ability stemmed from a stroke rather than the result of nerve damage. The hypertension in combination with the hardening of the arteries in the brain is an invitation for strokes to occur.

None of this should have been surprising. The natural course of aging produces hardening of the arteries in the brain, and the resulting high blood pressure would make sense. The chronic pulmonary condition could have been predicted from her many years of smoking.

There was, however, something awful for me in knowing these additional diagnoses. Before this medical meeting, I felt like all we were battling here was Alzheimer's.

I was shocked to realize I still held onto the hope she would recover and be whole enough to go out shopping with me on a Saturday morning, cruising yard sales, buying dolls, talking and laughing. But I did. Because she was still alive. She was still my mother. And my mother used to do those things.

For Lolly, the meeting with the medical personnel and the additional medical information was a relief. She felt she could at last accept there was something medically wrong with Mom. Mom was not just mean or crazy, but physically sick.

A terrible ambiguity surrounds Alzheimer's. Despite the number of physical and psychological tests used to reach the tentative conclusion someone might have Alzheimer's, you're always left wondering if the doctors might be wrong in their diagnosis. They are the first to admit the only REAL test for the disease is an autopsy.

So, you wonder if your loved one really does have Alzheimer's, or if the doctors have missed something. Maybe it isn't Alzheimer's at all, but a brain tumor, a vitamin deficiency, or some psychotic behavior, easily cured with a miracle drug like Prozac. Worse yet, you are left wondering if your mother isn't just a hateful old person who doesn't remember the good times or anything about her life or yours. The bottom line in all of this is: you wonder if somehow you've all failed to see the truth.

The new knowledge I now had that my mother possessed some real physical quirks and manifestations of both normal aging and Alzheimer's felt like a burden. The truth had at last been revealed: she could die from Alzheimer's, probably from some failure to swallow, drowning in her own spit, and she could also have a stroke and die. In fact, she had probably had a small stroke already.

The knowledge made me feel responsible. What were we to do with this knowledge? Demand preventative medication? But, what medication? Why? Have them alter her diet? To what? Something that lessened the hardening of the arteries in the brain? Something that would humanely speed the process? More chocolate, less chocolate, red wine, champagne?

We had once believed it would be a blessing if Mom had a stroke. Knowing it was a possibility, it no longer felt like a blessing. It felt confusing and awful and frightening. Mom does not know what is happening to her. I can't imagine how they even managed to calm her enough to get a blood sample from her or fasten a blood pressure cuff around her arm.

I thought of a friend whose mother recently died of cancer. She knew her mother was dying. Her mother knew she was dying, and together they planned a trip. It was a physically and emotionally hard trip. But, it was something they did together.

My mother and I cannot sit and make plans together. We cannot take a trip. We can't even cruise around some sunny Saturday afternoon looking for yard sales.

My brothers and sister and I visit. We wait. We talk to Mom and listen to her and wonder if she knows she is losing bits and pieces of her mind. We worry she knows she is slowly being ravaged and destroyed by something, most probably Alzheimer's.

There was an article in the paper the other day about a local blue grass performer who has bowed out of the concert circuit because he has Alzheimer's. I read the article with fascination. He clearly and lucidly described the episodes of memory loss he was experiencing: the blankness, the inability to call up lyrics he has sung for more than twenty years, putting a name and a face together on a friend, remembering what he has just done.

After reading the article, I wanted to ask Mom if she had these experiences. I wanted to know what it felt like for her. But I can't ask because she doesn't know. She isn't able to remember, and she never told us anything about how she felt until it was too late.

The week before, in a different article, a daughter recounted her mother's insistence, before it was discovered she had Alzheimer's, that she didn't want to hear anything bad. Mom did a similar thing. From about 1989 on, she didn't want to hear anything bad about our lives, but she became fascinated with grisly murders and cut out articles from the paper and carried them around in her purse. Once, when the children and I were sitting on the floor playing with blocks in Lolly's family room, Mom came in, sat down, opened her purse, and began reading aloud from one of these articles. When I tried to tell her I thought the incident was terrible, but not appropriate for the children to hear, she got mad and stormed out of the room. We were unable to talk about what she was thinking, why she read the article to me, why she carried it in her purse, or what she was afraid of or angry about.

We have no evidence she ever had a time where she knew what was happening to her and could think about what it meant. We are left believing she never had the chance to make plans or decisions for the rest of her life like this blue grass player. She never talked to us about what she felt or what she wanted.

Knowing her body is poised to have a stroke at any moment saddens me in a deep and disturbing way.

It doesn't seem right. None of this seems right. A stroke seems violent, a last wrenching of life. Let her sleep. Let her dream. Let her remember for a minute in the dream that she was once alive. Let her have a moment of peace slipping from one life to another.

CHAPTER ELEVEN

CHRISTMAS 1994

EARLIER IN THE FALL WE DECIDED WE WOULD BE ON OUR own for Thanksgiving, but would go up to Michigan to see Mom for Christmas. Jeff and I also decided we didn't want to drive. It is, even in the best of weather, a long drive, and neither of us finds driving a relaxing sport.

When we started to make plane reservations, the kids protested. They didn't want to fly. They weren't afraid of flying, but they also weren't in favor of flying. We wondered why. After several dinner discussions about what we were going to do, it came out the children felt flying was too abrupt, too sudden a wrenching from here to there. When I thought about it, I agreed.

It is hard to go "from here to there." The distance from our lives to Mom's is an ever-increasingly more difficult and distant trip. We didn't need transportation as much as we needed a way to ease into her life.

We chose the train, took full advantage of our five-hour layover in Washington, DC, going to the National Gallery's East Wing for lunch and browsing through both the Toulouse-Lautrec and Milton Avery shows before reboarding the train in time to make dinner reservations in the dining car. It is the most civilized way to travel.

Shortly after we pulled into Ann Arbor the next morning, we took Lolly to work and the kids to see Mom.

Mom was in the dining area of the medical wing eating lunch when we arrived. It was the first time we had been to see her since she had been moved two and a half months earlier.

Although clean and well cared for, the medical unit is not as visually appealing as Wesley Hall, the Alzheimer's floor. The halls are wider and barer in order to accommodate wheelchairs. There's a nurses' station at the center of the wing, and there's more medical support equipment, quietly signaling people here are impaired. Almost everyone is in a wheelchair or uses some sort of walking device. Most of the residents need assistance eating, so mealtimes are messy and take forever.

The overall impact of seeing Mom sitting alone in a wheelchair, a tray table with her lunch pulled close to her chair so she could work through trying to feed herself, while all around her, bibbed adults were being spoon-fed by attendants, was upsetting.

Lolly had said we would be shocked. The need for the wheelchair had dramatically changed Mom's appearance. Her inability to move independently robbed her of some of her fire. She didn't look up when we approached.

It took several minutes before she realized we were standing there speaking to her. Even then, she did not immediately respond to us or realize we were there for her.

When I sat down next to her to talk with her face to face, I noticed she was holding a doll. When I mentioned the doll, she stopped eating, took the doll in both hands and held it out at arm's length and began talking to it.

She talked, cooed, whistled, and made faces at the doll, rocking it back and forth so its eyes opened and closed. Then, she brought it close to her and held it on her shoulder like a baby and resumed eating. We stayed with her in the dining room until she finished her lunch then wheeled her out into the hall.

The dining room made me uncomfortable. I wanted to get out of there. Also, the youngest children, Cole and Colin, were proving dangerous with all the walkers and wheelchairs around, so we asked the attendant at the nurses' station if we could take Mom off the ward for a walk. She said yes, and explained Mom had on an alarm band, so we would need to trip the alarm device near the door in order to get out.

Getting out was not so easy. Mom, although she was in a wheelchair, was situated so her feet were resting on the floor. By shuffling her feet, she could propel the wheelchair forwards and backwards. She could also put her feet down stubbornly and stop you from moving her.

After some cajoling, coaxing, and gentle pushing, we got her going forward. Neil took charge of pushing Mom off the ward into the other areas of the building, while Jeff, the other kids, and I kept chatting away, pointing out all the nice things to see so we could keep her going through the halls.

It took awhile, but we moved through the building to the new wing where there is a sunny common seating area and an ice cream parlor. The ice cream parlor is run by volunteer residents who open it each afternoon from two to four, serving malts, shakes, sundaes, and sodas at minimal cost.

While we were waiting for the shop to open, we moved around the big sunny lobby area looking at the various Christmas decorations, trying to engage Mom in conversation. It was clear her language skills had declined, but she was oddly happier than we had seen her before. The doll seemed to calm her, and from time to time, she would take it from her shoulder and make faces at it, cooing and whistling, the way we all do when we are holding newborn babies.

By the time we finished our ice cream, maneuvered our way through the halls back to her new home, I was exhausted. It was a struggle to establish and maintain "contact" with her. The disease seemed to have come again in the middle of the night and robbed her of something new, some subtle piece of herself more essential than fine motor control, memory, or language.

The ancient Greeks believed the body had humors. Although the idea seems more mystically than medically sound, I wonder if the Greeks were right and if the Alzheimer's has boldly moved forward and robbed her of one of her essential humors. Even more horrifying: perhaps the disease has drained all it can from her memory and is now working its way through her soul. It takes all the inner strength I can muster to keep from screaming.

As I struggle to engage her, I feel as though I am also struggling to establish and maintain my own precarious sanity.

The next day. We leave the kids at home, so Lolly and I can go alone to visit Mom. When we get there, Mom seems agitated, distracted, and unfocused. I notice all the patients are parked in the hallway and two nurses are working their way from one end of the ward to the other. One of them approaches us.

"The doll is gone," she says, as though we know what she's talking about, "we can't find her doll. The doll really helps her. Did she have it when you came back yesterday?"

She did. I have a sudden chilling fear the doll might be her last connection with the world. Yes, the doll is important. We take Mom down the hall to her room. Calmly and methodically, we search the place. We check drawers, under the bed, the closet, the bathroom, the trash can, the little bookcase, behind the pillows in her chair. She has lost other things including her glasses, her teeth, and numerous purses and favorite gaudy necklaces. Many of these items have never been found and make me wonder if Alzheimer's doesn't have something to do with the mysterious black holes of the universe.

In our search, we take the time to look through her clothes. They're looking pretty laundry abused and shop worn. We decide we need to buy her some new things. Pretty things to make her look nice. We don't find the doll.

We had stopped by Mom's favorite bakery before we came and bought her three jelly donuts. She sees the box, and, like a child, her eyes light up and she becomes excited. When we give it to her, she opens it and starts in on the donuts. She is delighted, and enthusiastically licks jelly off her fingers as she moves from one donut to the next. The sugar from the donuts gets everywhere, and when we clean her up, washing her hands, her face, brushing the crumbs from her clothes, we take the opportunity to brush her hair, clean her up a little special. I enjoy the brief moment of doing and fussing, washing a small spot from her clothes, making her look nice. It is one of the only moments I have had recently where I feel as though being there with her matters.

We stay and visit for nearly two hours. Mostly, we sit with her, trying, when we can, to pick up and respond to what she is attempting to say. We tell her about her brothers and sisters and read their messages to her on the Christmas cards she's gotten, but when we ask her if she remembers her siblings, she gets distracted and visibly upset. I feel guilty we have never told her two of her sisters, Alice and Nedra, have died.

The staff still hasn't found the doll by the time we leave. We tell them we'll go and buy another one. The nurse at the desk brightens. "It's a help, really a help," she says, punctuating her words with her hands. She tells us Mom doesn't cry as much when she has the doll.

"The doll," she says, her face hopeful that we'll find what Mom needs, "has to have hair, and eyes that open and shut when you lay it down and pick it up, and hands," she holds her hands out like a child's, "that are curved, like this, with the fingers open. She tries to put things in the doll's hands, to feed it. And a nice face. The doll should have a nice face."

We leave the hospital to go shopping. It is Christmas Eve. We still have stockings to fill, presents to wrap, and dinner to cook. We're painfully aware we might not find this doll this late and so close to Christmas.

We go to a local discount store and work our way down the toy aisle, picking up boxes to see if eyes open and shut. We find a few, some with hair, some without, and begin to unbox those with hair to test them. We know a good doll has to be soft and easy to hold.

We quickly reject two with nice faces and fairly decent heads of hair because they are hard and cold to the feel. We check the hands and find a couple with nicely curled fingers and open palms.

In the end, we settle on a classic: a blond-haired, blue-eyed Betsy Wetsy with a wide face and smile. It's a good doll. She's dressed in a short top, matching booties, diaper and rubber pants. She has a comb and brush and a bottle. When the bottle is filled with water, it can be fed to the doll, and, as the name implies, this water works its way down to a wet diaper. The doll looks a lot like the one she lost. We think she'll like it.

Christmas Day. The kids are up early. The little ones are so excited by their stockings they don't even notice the unwrapped "Santa" presents waiting under the tree.

Charles came Christmas Eve and had dinner and then spent the night. It is fun having him here, like a big kid, waiting for Christmas. The kids have made a stocking for him filled with dozens of wrapped screwdrivers and small tools Lolly and Tom bought for him. They have fun watching him unwrap them.

We take our time opening the presents in turns, unwrapping the gifts one at a time, stopping on occasion to assemble something and play with it.

Once the gifts are undone and the paper is cleaned up, we go to the kitchen and work a little on the dinner preparations. With the turkey in the oven, we get ready to go see Mom.

It will be the first Christmas we don't bring her home. It feels odd and uncomfortable. The wheel-

chair and her lack of mobility, coupled with her growing unpredictability, have made it not only unwieldy,
but unwise to bring her home.

Colin is undone by all the excitement and desperate for a nap, so we leave Lolly and Colin at home
when we go. It is cold outside, but there isn't even a
hint of snow: another sign Christmas isn't right this year.

I'm surprised by how few cars there are in the
parking lot at the Methodist Home. I would have
thought there would be lots of families visiting or many
of the residents gone. But neither is true. It feels
like a regular day on the floor. Everyone present, ac-
counted for, and cruising along in their wheelchairs
and walkers.

We look for Mom but can't find her at first because she is still eating lunch in the dining area. We
wait while she finishes, then take her to the hall. A
nurse sees us carrying presents and pushing Mom. She
ushers us into a private sitting room and says we should
feel free to close the doors and stay there for as long
as we like. There don't seem to be too many other
families looking for places to visit.

The kids take off their coats and pile them up
on a chair. They are anxious for Mom to unwrap her
presents, for her to see her doll. It feels like Christmas for them again, but it takes Mom a long time to
understand she is supposed to unwrap the presents
the children give her. Cole is dancing around in front
of her, jiggling with excitement. He loves to help
unwrap things but always wants to try to save the paper. The wrapping paper has reindeer leaping across
a field of bright red and holly. The present is tied
with dozens of curled ribbons. Mom touches the bow
as if it is her present. Cole can't wait any longer and
shows her where the tape is easiest to pull off.

When the doll is uncovered, Mom seems pleased, but disconcerted it is trapped in the box. We pull it out to find it is held in place by long twist ties, and we work as fast as we can to get them undone because she is upset the doll can't move.

When I finally get the doll out, she won't look at it or take it. The kids are upset by her reaction and try to tell her the baby doll is hers. When she finally takes the doll in her hands, she tips it so its eyes will open and close. She talks baby talk to it, whistles to it, and makes odd clucking noises.

It is scary to witness your mother go through these gestures. Charles has pulled away from the group and is sitting back watching, tears rolling down his face.

We stay for about two hours, combing the doll's hair, talking to Mom, sitting with her, showing her the little plastic baby bottle so she can feed her doll.

Cole and Hedy wonder what the body of the doll looks like and try to take its clothes off. Mom waves her hands at them and warns them to be careful.

We are very careful. The day feels fragile, fractured, nearly destroyed. When it seems as though all the air has been sucked from the room we have been sitting in, we get our coats and start to go. We bring Mom out in the hall to say good-bye and let the nurse know we are going. Mom holds her doll on her shoulder, lifting it up from time to time to blow in its face, whistling at it, making its eyes blink as she rocks its body to and fro. The kids hug her and kiss her good-bye.

When we go down the hall, she tries to follow us. The nurse from the front desk comes to see the doll, to help us leave. Unexpectedly, as she is moving Mom down the hall, the nurse calls out to us, "Why wouldn't she want to follow you?" I feel scalded by her words, reproached for not being a good enough daughter to take my mother home for Christmas dinner.

We do not talk about Mom at all after we leave. Balancing our "well" lives against our mother's disease-riddled one is a terrible strain.

The day after Christmas. We need a mission, a purpose, so we dress to brave the biggest shopping/exchange day of the year to go in search of new things for Mom to wear. It feels like an adventure, a welcome release from a scary claustrophobic time.

Lolly has to work, so Tom, Jeff, and I have the kids. Neil and Quentin want to wander off on their own at the mall, which is fine. Tom and Jeff offer to take the two little ones exploring while Hedy and I shop for Mom.

We go to Lane Bryant. Mom, although she's smaller than she used to be, is still on the big side. We have to guess at her clothing size.

The wheelchair presents a number of clothing problems. Mom likes jackets and vests, but if they're too long, they're hard to sit in and wind up bunching up in the back and just being so much twisted material.

Everything is on sale and we decide to do it up right, getting her matching slacks and tops, a vest she can wear with several things, new pajamas and a robe.

Hedy and I have fun picking colors, matching outfits, and imagining what Mom would have picked out on her own. We talk about things looking "like grandma," and find things she might have thought were too expensive but would make her look smart. We are conscious we want her to look her best, to look like she is loved. We buy only those things we think are beautiful.

We pick the softest and prettiest long terry cloth robe we can find. The "tub" room is off the entrance hall of the ward. We want her to look good when she's out there waiting for her bath. We want her to feel wrapped up and warm when she finishes.

We are pleased with our purchases. When we go to visit her later in the afternoon, we do not give them to her, but to the attendant at the nurses' station so her name labels can be sewn into them, marking them for the laundry. The attendant remarks on how many things we've bought. We tell her we want Mom to look nice. When the tags are in, we'll go through her closet and get rid of those things too worn to be nice anymore. The wheelchairs and walkers of the medical wing work to reduce these residents to the category of patient. The shift of person to patient robs them all of some of their identity. The wealth of clothes we have purchased for Mom seems extreme to the attendant: it seems necessary to me. I want Mom to look great, to be a bit of sparkle in this otherwise drab existence. If she sparkles, maybe she'll be noticed more. Maybe someone will stop and compliment her, smile at her, make her feel like a person.

Again, we take Mom and the kids for a walk through halls of the complex and go "out" for ice cream. Everyone gets malts, including Mom, and the kids show her how to suck it up with a straw. Several times, she stops when she is drinking, to tell them it's good. She loves ice cream.

There is another family "out" for ice cream. They recognize Mom and say hello. Their mother is a patient on the Alzheimer's wing, Wesley Hall. They ask how it is where Mom is now. We tell them the truth: it is nice, but not as nice as Wesley. There's nothing else to say.

When we walk back through the building, we stop in the music room. Both Neil and Hedy sit down and play the organ for her. Because the organ faces a wall, their backs are facing her when they sit to play. Mom gets confused by the sound and doesn't realize they are playing for her.

When Neil is finished and Hedy takes her turn at the keyboard, Mom moves a little in her chair to watch what she is going to do. "Beautiful hands she has," Mom says, pointing at Hedy. It is the most appropriate and complete sentence she has made during the visit. Hedy does have beautiful hands, and Mom's statement catches me unprepared and makes me choke a little.

On our way back to Mom's room, we see an attendant from Wesley Hall, she stops to talk to Mom and to ask us how she's doing. We tell her she's declined. She says she's heard. She touches Mom's hand and tells her she misses her. I tell her it's all very sad and she agrees.

December 27. Colin and Quentin decide to stay home so Jeff and I just take Neil, Hedy, and Cole to see Mom. Lolly has to go to work again but suggests we take something to the hospital with us to "play" with Mom. She had tried the other week to color with her in a coloring book and had some success and thinks it might be good if we can get her to do something with her hands.

We decide on Play-Doh, so we stop at a couple of stores on our way to the Methodist Home. The shelves have pretty much been picked clean by Christmas. The only thing I find is a Play-Doh finger-puppet kit, so I buy it.

When we get to Mom's, things feel rocky. She doesn't recognize us and is very agitated we have come. She points at the kids and asks why they are there. I'm apprehensive about staying, but I don't know what else to do. At least with the Play-Doh in hand, the kids will have something to keep them busy while I try to talk with her and calm her.

Neil keeps trying to engage her with the Play-Doh, but she keeps pushing him away and saying, "No, no." I am playing with Neil and Hedy, pressing Play-Doh into the puppet forms around their fingers making little finger puppets of Elmo, Cookie Monster, Bert, and Ernie. Mom holds her doll close to her, stroking the back of its head, talking to it, holding it up above her head, and telling it what a good baby it is, one that has never given her trouble. I wish I knew what was going on in her mind.

I look up and realize Neil is gone. I get a little scared. I didn't see him go and hope he is all right. When he comes back, he doesn't come into the room but stands in the doorway.

He tells me he has heard a violin somewhere. Neil has played the violin since he was in third grade. He asks if he can find where the music is coming from. I tell him it's fine.

When he comes back, he is very excited. There's a man playing the violin in the dining room. He wants to take Mom. We gather up the Play-Doh and puppet forms and put them back into the box. Then we take Mom down the hall to hear the music.

The attendants are wheeling people into the dining room. There's a woman playing the piano and a man strolling around the room playing a violin. One of the residents is clapping his hands and singing. The others sit and listen and watch or doze.

When the man stops, Neil approaches him and asks if he can borrow his violin for a moment. The man hands it to him and Neil faces Mom and starts to play. He plays bits and pieces from his recent recital and a few pieces he has performed with his orchestra at middle school. Neil is good and has always played in a way you don't expect a child to play, as though it is part of his heart. The man is surprised, even more surprised when he finds out our six-foot-one Neil is only thirteen.

For the next forty-five minutes Neil and the man, a local Methodist minister who comes every week to play for them, take turns playing. It is a natural and easy exchange, the violin trading hands every couple of songs. The man nearest the piano claps his hands loudly and sings, hardly noting the switch of players, while the others sit and watch.

Once or twice Mom looks at Neil when he plays, but the look is more puzzling than praising. She seems unsure the music is coming from him. She watches him, then looks away, then turns back and watches again, but mostly, she fiddles with her doll and strokes its hair.

When it's time for us to leave, Mom fusses a little with the doll, straightening her clothes and moving her arms. The kids take turns touching Mom and saying good-bye. She doesn't attempt to follow, and in fact, hardly notices when we go.

December 29. We take a brief "vacation" day in Lansing, playing with the kids at the hands-on science museum, the Oldsmobile museum, and the newly refurbished state capitol. It is just the break we need to get our balance back and believe we are a family again.

December 30. Now that Mom is on a medical unit, care meetings are scheduled every ninety days for the staff to report to the family. Since it is time for another meeting, we go ahead and schedule one so both Lolly and I can attend.

The meetings are held off the ward in a conference room on the first floor. One of the nurses attends as well as the program director. Although the meeting is supposed to be informal and purely for information purposes, my stomach feels as though we have been called to the principal's office.

At Lolly's first meeting she had to sign off on the level of care we wanted them to pursue: i.e., how much medical intervention we wanted on Mom's behalf. The options are reviewed, and, again, we choose "Code A," indicating we want Mom to be comfortable; if necessary, she should be treated with antibiotics for infections and narcotics for pain; we do not want her transferred to an intensive care setting; and we want no aggressive treatment or life supports. We have not changed our thinking. Without any hesitation, all four of us, her children, have agreed this is what she would want, but having to review the options a second time, in the context of the hospital, is creepy.

I remind myself, over and over again in my head, this is what I would want for myself. In fact, I wonder sometimes if we have already done too much, pushed and prolonged her life too far with the seemingly benign yet gentle intervention of placing her in the care of the Methodist Home. I don't know anymore if I would want to live at all without a mind. I do not know if I could live half knowing, half not knowing my children would have to watch me deteriorate memory by memory, capability by capability. When I think of my mother's present life, I feel the urge to live dangerously, take risks, drink a tad more champagne than is good for me, eat chocolate, and hope if I am genetically destined to get Alzheimer's, I will get lucky enough to die from some foolishness devised by my own hand, full of life, not drained of it.

The meeting feels uncomfortably serious. The staff is thorough and caring. They review Mom's blood pressure, her recent weight gain, her charted problems of cerebral arteriosclerosis, hypertension, pulmonary lung problems from years of smoking cigarettes, and her recent change and increase of medication. She is now on Pazil and Mellavil, antidepressants and antianxiety drugs, and seems to be responding better. They mention the doll and note they are unsure what is responsible for her recent move from deep depression to manageable depression: the drugs or the doll, or the two in tandem.

They talk about her meeting her "goals." I want to giggle, but suppress the urge. Mom hasn't got a clue she has "goals" she is expected to meet. The staff, however, is quite serious about these goals, and, although the idea seems silly, I realize these goals keep the staff focused on her care, keep them encouraged and working to help her. I am grateful they can hold tight to such an idea.

One completed goal they discuss with pride is reducing her crying to two hours or less a day. My heart is drained and I want to cry myself. They are thrilled to report she has reached her goal and, with the help of the doll, no longer sits outside the director's office crying all day.

We ask about visiting her. We want to know if it helps. We are looking less for the truth than a reassurance we are doing something right or need to do it more often, because we are so unsure ourselves. Sometimes it feels right. Sometimes it feels awful. She is unable to verbalize how she feels and we leave not knowing if our coming has been good or bad. More often than not, we are at an emotional loss as to what we should do, and we are embarrassed by our lack of knowledge and understanding regarding what is good for our mother.

Oddly enough, the staff shift in their chairs a little: they are the ones uncomfortable with the question. The truth: since we have been visiting every day this week, Mom has been more difficult, more agitated and volatile. There have been a couple of incidents, difficult times for the staff, when she has lashed out. Morally, it is right to visit, management-wise, it is difficult if we come. My head spins. I have lost some thread, the reality of what a family is, what constitutes relationships and responsibilities, how to recognize and work toward some goal of mutual happiness.

We ask, remembering the comment the staff member made to us regarding Mom's desire to follow us out the door, if we should try to take her out again. The idea sounds like a good one, but on second thought, the staff is unsure how long Mom can be gone and not become confused and overwhelmed, scared and violent.

I am beginning to understand the security of staying with "goals," of focusing on things like blood pressure, weight gain and loss, and medicine dosage. Pressed with anything so weighty as obligation and relationships, we snap like taut rubberbands and begin to focus on maintenance details: they've added side rails to her bed, she needs to have some minor medical procedures and tests done, and we have to sign papers approving IV sedation.

I mention noticing there is always a carton of milk on her meal tray. I tell them Mom has never in her life willingly drunk a glass of milk. I tell them I suspect she is lactose intolerant and want it noted in her chart. If they force her to drink milk, she'll have trouble with her stomach and will also become unwilling to eat and will wind up having to be force-fed: something we want to avoid. I make the observation on her behalf, hoping to gain some dignity for her, some sense of choice.

The nurse stiffens. She wants to know how I propose Mom will get her daily calcium requirement. I suggest she can get it through puddings, cheese, ice cream, or even tablets.

Since we brought it up, the nurse wants to discuss our taking Mom to the ice cream parlor. During her last medical workup it was discovered she has an elevated cholesterol. I cannot help myself. I sharply blurt out that most postmenopausal women have elevated cholesterols. The nurse ignores me and continues her lecture.

She notes Mom has gained ten pounds in the past three months. We note she lost forty in the previous two years during which time she was agitated, active, and prowling the halls. Since she is now confined to a wheelchair, we suggest a ten-pound weight gain would seem natural.

While she's at it, the nurse says she doesn't want us to bring Mom jelly donuts anymore. She wants us to substitute jelly beans instead. I bite my tongue.

While we sit ever so still, the nurse waxes on about lowfat sweet options, cholesterol, and high blood pressure problems. She has become the guardian of Mom's glowing health. She cannot see the forest for the trees: there is no earthly reason to deny Mom anything, not ice cream, jelly donuts, chocolate, or if she asked for it, salted peanuts, beer, and cigarettes.

Lolly and I look at each other and know there is no need to pursue this line of reasoning, no converts to be made: the ice cream and donuts will continue. We have learned to pick our fights.

I mention we want to have Mom's eyes examined. We are worried she might be developing cataracts again. Her right eye is tearing pretty much all the time. The first time she had the cataracts removed they were diagnosed as "juvenile." We were told the "adult" variety might develop later. We also want her to be seen by a dentist. We want her to have a new set of false teeth made to replace the ones she lost.

The director and the nurse make a note in their charts and begin to talk about scheduling appointments. The nurse seems satisfied to have something to add to her set of goals and objectives.

"This is good," she says, "these things should be done, need to be done. After all, your mother is only seventy-five. She could easily live another twenty years."

I feel the impact of her statement like a truck hitting me broadside. My sister puts her hand on the edge of the table to steady herself.

Twenty more years. I cannot, do not, hear anything else that is said. Then we get up and go in silence. It's time to meet the kids, Jeff, and Tom and then go upstairs to see Mom.

We meet them coming in the door and go up the elevator together. Mom is in the dining room sitting with her friend, Penny. Penny has a new doll too, and the two of them are sitting at a table, jabbering, and playing with their dolls. An attendant comes in with one of those mechanical parrots with a tape recorder inside that repeats what you say. She uses it to help the patients with their language skills. The kids have fun playing with it. Mom and Penny watch intently, holding onto their dolls.

While we are visiting, a sermon begins to be broadcast over the loudspeakers. It is Friday afternoon, an odd time for a sermon, and we listen curiously. We quickly realize we are listening to a funeral service for one of the residents who must have died over Christmas.

The attendants are wheeling in residents. We don't know if they are bringing them into the dining room to get them ready to eat lunch, or if they are bringing them here to listen to the service. The kids have quit playing with the parrot and are focused on the broadcast. I do not want them listening. I do not want them thinking about dying this Christmas. I do not want them to be burdened any longer with the weight of all these damaged lives at the Methodist Home, or of their grandmother whom they adore, falling apart, falling out of life, out of their lives, without a chance or a clue.

I hear the declaration of the nurse ringing in my ears: "She could live another twenty years."

The broadcast is too cruel, too bizarre. I want it to end. We wheel Mom out of the dining room, down the hall to her room, to get her away. We all need to escape.

We fuss a little over Mom in her room and comb her hair. We look out the window and talk about the possibility of snow. We tell Mom we will come back in the spring, when the flowers are coming up, to see her again. She seems connected for a moment.

We walk Mom down to the dining room, hoping we have stayed away long enough for the funeral service to be over. I do not want her to have to eat lunch listening to the service. The room is quiet except for the noise of the patients and the unloading of lunch trays. We do not go in, but stay instead in the hallway, saying our good-byes. The kids give her hugs. Neil touches her head and says good-bye. I kiss her cheek and try to look at her eye to eye, hoping she'll understand I have to go but will come back soon. Mom doesn't seem to notice we are leaving and takes her doll and begins to coo and whistle at it again.

When we get to the parking lot, the kids go with Tom and Jeff and Lolly and I get into her car. We don't even try to speak until both doors are firmly closed against the cold.

"Twenty years," Lolly says, her hands braced against the steering wheel, "my life is over."

A dark thick depression begins to take hold. We try to chase it off, laughing about the jelly donuts, making a pact we will never come again without donuts in hand.

Mom should have donuts. She should have something to look forward to, something that brings her joy. And we should have our lives, but our lives are caught for this moment in time with hers and we are drowning with her. We can't talk about what we are thinking: that we believe she is already dead and we need to give up trying to swim with her to shore; that we need to let go of her; that she would not want to prolong her life if she knew her mind was wasted; and that twenty more years like this seems like a black and lifeless eternity.

"I mean it, Carrie," my sister says, starting the car and putting it in reverse, "I'm going to get a gun, and if I get this disease, I'm going to go out into the woods, and I'm going to shoot myself."

When we get home, I cannot tell Jeff what happened during the care meeting. I cannot articulate the sadness, pain, and frustration I feel. I shut down. I spend the afternoon packing our suitcases. I cannot talk. I cannot say anything.

When we are in the kitchen, cleaning up from dinner, getting ready to go to the train station, I tell my sister I have only spent three Christmas vacations in my life in my own home. It is the wrong thing to say, but I can't help myself. It is not her fault. She reminds me I am the one who moved away. She stayed. She lives with this every day.

I am sorry. I am overwhelmed with this burden, this half-life, and feel responsible, for what, I no longer know. I want to make it better. I want to take my sister away, to give her a break. I want my mother to wake up one morning and be well enough to fly to my house and live with me and play with my children.

I want to run away. I want all of this to be done with and gone, and yet, I know I can't escape. I also know, even though I will get on a train, ride through the night to get home the next day, I will not be able to get far enough away to have my own life.

I feel selfish. I feel angry. I feel overwhelmed with all this disease means for our lives.

CHAPTER TWELVE

FEBRUARY 1995

AN IMPASSIONED YOUNG WOMAN IN A TIGHT BLACK DRESS takes the podium at the Ninth Annual Joseph and Kathleen Bryan Alzheimer's Disease Research Center Conference. She is the first speaker on the program. She claims she's nervous but looks out into the audience in a self-assured, uncocky way I will grow to appreciate as the conference unrolls. She's here to tell her mother's story. Her mother, she says, slowing her speech and looking out over our heads to the back of the room, was diagnosed with Alzheimer's two years ago when she was forty-seven years old.

The shock of her statement jolts us awake. Forty-seven. The number murmurs through the crowd like a strong current, a wave gathering momentum to break. We listen, knowing how the story will unravel, because many people in the crowded room have lived the story, have had the phone calls, watched the decline, struggled with the financial, physical, philosophical, and psychological burden of it all. We know.

She has more to say. She is here for a reason. She wants everyone, every doctor, every researcher, social worker, preacher, teacher, mother, and daughter, to know her mother was not dumb. She uses the word "dumb" like a hammer as she reels off her mother's academic and career accomplishments. It's an impressive list. Her mother was working as the president of a company when she was diagnosed with Alzheimer's. She's telling her mother's story because she wants to put a stop to the demoralizing, damaging, and blatantly false assumption both doctors and researchers are working from that if you have a bright active mind you won't get Alzheimer's.

I feel the crowd of caretakers wanting to rise to their feet and applaud. The shared sentiment is palpable. There is hope in this room. We are here to share, to learn, and to push the falsehoods aside in order to move forward in this awful business.

Afterwards, before we break for lunch, an expert, someone with a string of degrees and a title, gets up and rambles through her identified and published list of risk factors leading to Alzheimer's. There's barely a ripple of dissension when she takes her battery-operated flashlight pointer and circles "lower education" emblazoned on the screen before us, and tells us lower intelligence and lower education are both identified risk factors for Alzheimer's.

We are living in two worlds here: one of research, the other of reality. Someone grumbles over lunch that no one should be allowed to do research unless they have some firsthand experience of what they intend to study. Everyone at the table agrees that even good research done by bright well-meaning people, when done in the abstract, can be wrongheaded. Despite the discussion at lunch and my own feelings that research often misses the mark of reality, I'm feeling charitable. I am willing to brush off this little misfire of the morning and momentarily suspend judgment against this one researcher's work. I sense there is much to learn from the professionals here.

My mind races in renewed hope when another researcher begins her talk by commenting that she believes the "cure" for Alzheimer's will not be a single treatment, but a broad spectrum of treatments because the disease is a syndrome with multifactorial etiology. She speaks clearly and rationally about not only the tangle in the brain, but the tangle of the presenting symptoms and the complexity of addressing individual symptoms without adversely affecting others.

I am caught up in the mental exercise of seeing Alzheimer's as a puzzle, spread out on a table, some of the pieces lying face down, waiting for someone to turn them over to discover their fit. There is an excitement to this researcher's model that makes me feel like a cure is just sitting there waiting to be found. But, before I can cast off my discomfort with how little we presently know and can do about Alzheimer's and enjoy the possibilities this presenter's ideas bring forward in the disease model, another speaker brings me back on course.

He tells the story of a young medical student who had great promise and intelligence. This medical student was sitting at his desk one night studying, while his roommate practiced fencing in the room. At precisely the moment when the medical student turned

143

to watch, the roommate thrust the tip of his foil through the medical student's left eye into the memory center of his brain. He was left blinded in one eye and with no short- or long-term memory.

The tragedy of this lost "life" is overwhelming. I grieve quickly and deeply for the hell this young man is left to live in, and shake myself to realize this is the same hell my mother lives in now.

The roller coaster churns on. During the next session a hell-bent-for-leather-caught-up-in-his-own-corner-of-research physician pushes the professional care providers in the group to get signed consent for tube feeding early in the game so there aren't any "five-o'clock Friday" emergency orders begging for signatures. Nutrition and weight management is his concern, and, as he says, "with tube feeding, we can extend these people's lives another three to five years."

My blood pressure skyrockets. I want to scream. Would that young medical student, his lost colleague, want to be tube fed? Would he want another three to five years of not knowing, not remembering, not "living?"

My patience is gone. Now, like my fellow care-takers who grumbled over lunch, I want to put a halt to this conference. Research like this man's has fallen off the track. Someone should dial 911 and ask for the help of a philosopher, a theologian, or an ethicist. We've lost it.

There is an oddly surreal moment during the second day when Joseph Bryan is wheeled in to be honored. He is the benefactor of the conference, and of the Joseph and Kathleen Bryan Neurobiology Research Building at Duke University. It is his birthday. He is ninety-nine years old and the flat, blank expression

144

on his face hints that he might have some form of dementia. He has been brought forward for us to sing to him. There is a cake blazing with candles. One of the doctors from the Alzheimer's Disease Research Center at Duke is answering questions from the audience when Mr. Bryan is wheeled in. The doctor notes Joseph Bryan's entrance with a slight nod of his head, but keeps his back to the man and continues talking. Someone from the audience has asked a question regarding a recently published treatment for Alzheimer's that is not one of those under study by Duke's research team. The doctor's answer is snide. He seems to have forgotten, or rudely overlooked, the probability that the woman he is addressing is struggling with the reality that she fits the research "risk" profile. Her voice trembles and cracks when she repeats her question. She is not a doctor or a health professional. She is scared. More than likely, she is the primary caregiver for a parent suffering from Alzheimer's and knows firsthand what hell lies ahead.

The candles continue to burn while the doctor from Duke talks on. Mr. Bryan sits in his wheelchair, not noticing the candles or the speaker. Mr. Bryan is handsomely dressed. His vacant facial expression indicates he hasn't got a clue why he is here. When we stand to sing happy birthday to him, he sings along. The doctor who has berated the woman in the audience now blows out the candles for Mr. Bryan. They are trick candles and relight. The doctor laughs and blows again and again until he successfully extinguishes the flames. Mr. Bryan stares out blankly into the audience.

It is one of those horrible times when you are aware you know both too much and too little. The knowledge is uncomfortable. The situation is grotesque. I wrestle with getting my coat and leaving, but decide I have paid for this opportunity to learn something from these experts, these cutting-edge scientists, so I should stay, no matter how uncomfortable I feel right now.

The next session is beyond tedium. I do not blame the speaker but blame myself for staying. The speaker drones on and on about her concerns about weight loss in Alzheimer's patients.

My mother lost weight when she moved to the Alzheimer's wing. It seemed perfectly normal to us. She was eating a balanced diet devoid of her favorites: Doritos, cheeseburgers, fries, malts, Baby Ruths, and jelly donuts. She was also pacing the halls day and night. Why shouldn't she lose weight?

When she lost control of her right foot and had to use a wheelchair, she began gaining weight. This also seemed natural. All of a sudden, an active, almost hyperactive adult became sedentary, and her diet hadn't changed, so she gained weight.

I have no patience with this presentation and the researcher's silly scientific niggling. I stay through lunch to say good-bye to some of the people I have met, then beg off with the excuse I have to pick up the kids from the babysitter.

I am consumed by the packet of materials I have gathered from this conference. I feel as though my mother is with me, watching over my shoulder, looking for some cure, some relief from her pain. She is in my dreams and my waking thoughts. She pushes her way through the graphs and fancy projections of the probability of getting Alzheimer's. I can almost feel her hand grappling with the papers, trying to find the part of her that is missing.

She is in pain. It doesn't matter to her that anyone else might get this disease. It doesn't matter to her what the risk factors are or the probable causes. She is looking for more than a cure, she is looking for a balm, a way to ease her pain, to retrieve what she has lost, and to think clearly again. There are times now when I feel my mind has gone with hers. If her memory is lost, then so is my past. If her future cannot be grasped, than mine cannot either. We are tied by more than DNA and gene pools: we are tied by love, by history, by strong chords and bonds. She is my mother, I am her daughter. This obviously means more than these researchers have found.

The pathology of this disease is secondary to its path of destruction. We are, however, unable to realize the full impact of the destruction because of the clever packaging: old age. Which is precisely the reason the stories of the forty-seven-year-old mother and the medical student are so important. They are the "humanizing" stories of the disease. The shock of the realization that people who are not at the end of their lives, but in the middle, and therefore, should, like everyone else who has a future, have a memory, can and do get Alzheimer's, should shake us into thinking in new ways.

The medical student clears my mind. I try to visualize him when I think of my mother and what is best for her. The medical student cannot study and learn because he cannot remember what he has read. Likewise, movies make no sense. Friendships seem out of reach, because there is no recognition, no memory of past conversations or connections. A love relationship is almost impossible to imagine. As I try to use him as a model to understand what is happening to my mother a question nags at me: Does his lack of memory make him an imbecile?

Is memory intelligence? If it is, what is life like without intelligence?

As my mother loses mobility, the answer seems clear: put her in a wheelchair. But what about her mind? We do not have wheelchairs for minds. We have no artificial means to propel memory along or to make up for what is missing in someone's brain. Is there some computer aid we need to explore? Some memory tricks we haven't tried yet?

My mother is agitated and depressed. These are symptoms the medical professionals know how to treat: they medicate. They tried Prozac and a number of other drugs and finally hit on some combination to help her contain herself better. But, only better. She is not normal. She is not happy.

How can she be happy when nothing makes sense, when no moment connects to the next? The thread of her "life" is gone.

Like a researcher on a quest for a missing piece, I am consumed with trying to work out in my own mind the structure of this puzzle. I cannot sort out what is best for her. My gut reaction says tube feeding is inhumane: it denies her the taste of food, one of the few momentary pleasures she has left; it is a process and procedure she cannot understand, and it might also cause her some pain; and, foremost, forcing her to "eat" in this manner in order to sustain a life without a past or a future feels wrong. I know, without question, if I get Alzheimer's I do not want to be tube fed.

Two days after the conference, I am driving with some friends in a car. As we ride along, one of them tells a story about how her grandmother stayed alive long enough to see her mother one last time before she died. It is a moving and powerful story about the body's will to live for a connection to love and life. As she tells the story I can visualize this woman's mother driving through the night to see her mother, coming into the room around dawn, taking her mother's hand, telling her she loves her, knowing full well that her presence will enable her mother to take her last breath and die peacefully.

Ironically, this story sums up our dilemma: our mother no longer has anyone to wait for because she doesn't know us anymore. Just as she has died already for us, we have died for her. We are gone from each other's lives, but we are still living in each other's worlds.

I feel pressed by the conference I attended to look at new ways to make connections with my mother and for my mother with the world in general and the medical establishment specifically. This is really the task at hand.

I fear we are doing this business all wrong and need to rethink "treatment," and be more creative in our "medical management." We must spend both time and money to explore possible new pleasures and opportunities that are being missed for Alzheimer's victims and their families.

Alzheimer's claims many victims in its brushfire of destruction: family members are often as deeply burnt as the patients themselves. Sometimes, we wonder if we are the ones hurting, while Mom continues oblivious to her condition.

I understand weight gain and weight loss are significant indicators of disease and disorder in a body. I also understand there is more to Alzheimer's than body mass. Researchers need to talk with medical ethicists and with families in order to get a clear picture of what is at stake in the lives of all involved.

We also need to remember the stories of the promising medical student and young mother in order to shake ourselves free from the blinding concept that Alzheimer's is strictly a geriatric disease suitably treatable with a geriatric model.

CHAPTER THIRTEEN

SEPTEMBER 1995

MY BROTHER CHARLES WAS THE ONE TO CALL. I WAS GET-ting dinner ready when the phone rang. He was shaken but sounded calm. Mom had broken her hip. Despite the wheelchair, she had never quite understood her right leg didn't work anymore and she was unable to walk. She'd taken a couple of spills trying to get out of her wheelchair before, but, other than a bruise or two, had done herself no real harm until now.

Charles said he had talked to the Methodist Home, and Mom was on her way to St. Joseph's Hospital in Ann Arbor in an ambulance. I told him I'd call him back as soon as I could get a plane reservation.

It was too late to catch an evening flight, so I booked the first one out the next morning for Cole

151

and me. I called Charles to let him know Cole and I would be coming in the morning, then called Lolly at work to let her know when we'd be arriving.

The next morning, Lolly picked us up at the airport. We dropped our two boys off at Colin's nursery school, then drove straight to the hospital. When we arrived a little after 10 A.M., Mom was in preop and the surgeon was waiting for us. There were papers to sign. In our haste and confusion, we had forgotten Mom was no longer a consenting adult and that we would have to sign for her.

The nurse took us to see Mom. She was on a gurney with IVs running in the back of her hand and her right leg was bolstered by pillows. She was heavily sedated and didn't respond when we touched her or called out her name.

The nurse handed us a clipboard jammed with papers and told us to read them and sign in the appropriate places. The doctor would be over to see us directly and would discuss the operation with us. If we preferred, we could wait to sign until after we had talked to him.

There were many papers. The task was daunting, and the sudden escalation of responsibility was overwhelming. Lolly read through the first set of papers regarding the dangers of anesthesia and turned to me. The question was simple: What would Mom want?

It was THE question that had rumbled and rolled around in the air for the past five years. We had all thought about what she would want when it came to life supports, tube feeding, surgery, and medical interventions of any kind. Whenever we talked about it we all agreed, above all else, Mom was fiercely proud, and we knew without question she would want a life and a death with a sense of dignity.

But what, in the day to day of living and dying, does life and death with dignity really mean? Also, who Mom was before and who she is now are two different people. Even if the "old" mom could by some miracle come back for an hour to help us make decisions for her, we weren't sure she would know what this "new" mom would want.

The surgeon drew the curtain back and made a place for himself in our little circle and softly, clearly, laid out the options: 1) do nothing, 2) do a full hip replacement, or 3) pin the broken ball joint. We asked questions and he answered. He was candid and straightforward. Doing nothing would involve a lot of medication, waiting, and lying still. A full hip replacement would have to be followed by intensive physical therapy. Pinning the broken joint would be the least invasive surgery and would give her, in time, the same mobility she had before and would require only limited physical therapy.

When he finished his talk and answered our questions, he paused briefly before going on: no matter what our decision, and it was OUR decision as legal guardians, in his experience, when Alzheimer's victims suffered a physical trauma like a broken hip, they usually took some unexpected slide backwards, losing some ability. It might be motor, it might be cognitive, he didn't know. But he wanted us to be aware that although he could fix the hip, in some way, she would change. She would not be the same.

Not be the same as what? The Mom we knew was gone. The one that remained had become some rapidly flickering kaleidoscope of pieces falling and mating, scrambling and reassembling at random. Every day seemed to bring a new someone we didn't know any better than the last that had momentarily been in focus. The prospect of a dramatically diminished person now becoming "Mom" left us holding our breath.

"What do we do?" Lolly asked as the doctor stepped away to let us discuss the options. The doctor had carefully explained they could only do the full hip replacement if Mom were capable of physical therapy. When we asked what that entailed, he asked if she could follow directions. The answer was simple: no. That option was gone.

So, we were really down to two options: doing nothing and keeping her immobilized with medication until the hip could stabilize on its own, or doing the minimal surgery to pin the broken joint. Both of these options had their problems, but the bottom line was clear: we would be the ones to decide.

I thought I knew when we made the decision to put Mom in the Methodist Home what it was to make decisions for someone else. I thought my brothers and sister and I had felt the weight of that burden and had continued to shoulder the responsibility as she was moved from the Alzheimer's wing to the medical wing. Those early decisions, it turned out, were merely a warm-up, a little exercise in our growing responsibility for Mom.

Now, we would have to decide whether or not she would have surgery or be confined to bed and kept immobile with drugs. In order to clarify our own thinking, Lolly and I talked again about our decision at the Methodist Home to have Mom declared a Code A, i.e., no tube feeding, life supports, or resuscitation. We were quite clear on this issue. Even though Mom never made a living will, she made it clear to us, long before she had Alzheimer's, she did not want to be kept alive by any artificial means.

Would she want to be drugged and kept immobile in a bed in order to have her hip heal? Probably not. So, we made the only decision we thought reflected her wishes: to have her hip pinned.

When we talked to the doctor, giving him our decision, we explained her Code status and reviewed her history of Alzheimer's. He drew pictures of the surgical procedure and took time to answer more questions, then, before he left, he told us he thought we made the most humane decision, the same decision he would have made if she were his mother.

It took Mom a long time to come around after the surgery. Her breathing was erratic and labored and her blood pressure danced all around. We stayed with her until late in the evening when she, at last, stabilized.

The next morning she had a fever and the threat of pneumonia. Her blood count and blood pressure were dropping, so we had to sign more papers authorizing antibiotics and a couple of units of blood.

She was extremely agitated and went in and out of sleep, talking in both states of consciousness in a jumbled, crazy way, punctuated by shouts and threatening swipes of her hand. The staff informed us we were to let them know anytime we were leaving so they could put her in a straightjacket in order to keep her from pulling out her IVs.

The IVs were a problem. They bothered her. But there were other things that agitated her as well: the parade of nurses, blood pressure and temperature checks, and the long plastic inflatable cuffs on her legs that alternately pumped up and released first one leg then the other in order to prevent blood clots from forming in her legs. It was impossible to explain to her why they were there and what they did for her. Whenever she pulled at them and we moved her hands away and attempted once again to tell her they had to stay, she would shake her finger at us and shout, "No, no, no, you, you, you, don't."

Keeping her hands away from the IVs and the cuffs was exhausting. It was, however, easier to manage psychologically than having her constrained in a straightjacket.

We stayed with her for four days and on into the nights when she at last would fall into a deep, deep sleep. One day Colin and Cole went with me while Lolly went to work. Another day, just Cole came. The boys were a good distraction, although occasionally for no explainable reason she would start to shout at them, "No, no, no, you, you, you, don't."

When she slept she would have long disjointed conversations while her arms waved and reached out. During these times I began to wonder if there were spirits in the room.

One evening, waiting for her to fall into a peaceful state of sleep, I found myself wishing my mother's sister, Aunt Alice, her favorite of all her siblings, would come to visit her. Alice had died a couple of years before from cancer, and it seemed to me as though she was talking to Alice in these animated sleep conversations. Maybe she was.

One morning when I came to stay with Mom, a rather curt physical therapist informed me I had to leave because she was getting Mom up for a walk. When I asked her who was going to help her, she put her hands on her hips and informed me she didn't need anyone to help her.

I stood there dumbfounded. Mom hadn't walked for almost a year by then. She was also both big and strong and had a history of fighting with anyone who tried to move her physically.

"Did you see the chart?" I asked her. "Mom has Alzheimer's."

"Of course, but she can still walk."

"Who said?" I asked, this time getting a little annoyed.

"She did."

I was sure Mom did, because if anyone asked her anything, she would either say yes or no depending on her mood. At about this point in our conversation, the therapist pulled my mother's shoulders up from the bed in an attempt to sit her up. My mother started shouting, "No, no, no, you, you, you, no, no, no." Her voice was firm and commanding, and the fight in her eyes flashed wildly enough for the therapist to reconsider her intentions and ease Mom back down onto her pillows. The therapist then turned and left the room mumbling something about a person ought to know well enough if she can walk or not. The therapist never came back.

A couple of weeks before the fall that broke her hip, Mom had a fight with a gentleman on the ward. The staff was never able to discern what provoked the fight, but in the end, Mom and the man got in a tussle over his cane, and they both wound up on the floor. Mom suffered a bad bruise on her head and her glasses got broken. The man was a little bruised as well. Overall, Mom was very combative and it was not always possible to anticipate when she might feel like fighting. There were some times, however, when she would warn you.

One morning when I came to stay with her she was very angry. The IVs had been in for three days by then and must have been very uncomfortable. When

I walked into the room she turned her head away from me and started yelling, "No, no, no, you, you, you."

Then she held out her hand. When I moved forward to touch her, I began talking quietly about not being able to take out the IVs. This made her very agitated. She pulled her hand back and tried to pull the needle out on her own, so I gently, but quickly, took both her hands in mine and held them.

She calmed, then dropped her hands to her sides and started mumbling something that sounded distinctly like, "Slap you, slap you."

This seemed to me like a fair enough warning so I let go and backed off. Just as I was backing away, the new shift nurse came in. I had never met her before and introduced myself. She was one of those lovely-but-a-little-too-bubbly ladies in white.

"These Alzheimer's people are the sweetest old things," she gushed. And, before I could stop her she bent down over my mother's head to kiss her.

I could hear the pitch of my mother's voice rise as the woman moved closer to her, the cadence, "slap you, slap you," building steam. I could see what was going to happen. I had seen my mother hit a nurse before. I had no desire to witness it again, so I calmly told her to move back.

"Listen," I said, "she's saying she's going to slap you. Move back. She will. She's going to slap you."

It was an incredible relief to have Mom moved back to the Methodist Home where people knew her and respected her little idiosyncrasies. It was a relief to have the IVs gone and the pumping machine pulled off, as well as all the decision making over with for awhile.

As the doctor predicted, Mom did decline. Over the next couple of months following the surgery, she began to lose more language. By Christmas she had only twenty or thirty words left. No, yes, you, now, good, boy, need, don't, okay, are the ones that ring in my head.

In addition, no matter how hard the physical therapist at the Methodist Home would try, Mom refused to move her hurt leg. She would also, from time to time, start to cry and say the word "hurt."

To make matters much more complicated, she developed a fighting-mad phobia about being taken off the ward. It made sense to me. The last time they took her away, she went to a place that hurt her, kept her tied down, and poked her all the time. Her fear of being taken away from the ward, although a difficult situation, let us know she still made real-life connections in her mind. As complicated as this new development was, it reassured us "Mom" was still there.

Unfortunately, Mom had to be taken back to St. Joseph's for x-rays a couple of weeks later as a follow-up to the surgery. Lolly accompanied her. It took nearly four attendants to move Mom and keep her from hurting herself, and an additional corps of hospital personnel to get the x-rays. Lolly said it was an amazing three-hour battle. She was exhausted when she finally got Mom back to the Methodist Home.

By the time Christmas came around, I realized I too had reached a new plateau with the Alzheimer's: I was emotionally drained. I couldn't seem to get focused and get Christmas brewing at home. Lolly, however, was doing better. Between us there only seemed to be so much energy. Given that she was the one with the most pressing and immediate responsibility for Mom's care, I was glad she was rolling high.

Once again, we had reservations for the train to go to Michigan for Christmas. If nothing else, Alzheimer's had introduced us to train travel. The slow, leisurely, enforced relaxation of the train was wonderful for all of us. For the children it was an adventure punctuated by dinner in the dining car and a late-night movie in the observation car while the train rolled through the illuminated Christmas backyards of Virginia, Pennsylvania, and Ohio. For me it was the time to read, relax, and adjust to the reality that the Mom I was going to see would again be different from the last.

Flying was too abrupt, too sudden of a movement from here to there: from the sanity of our home to the craziness of Mom and the Methodist Home. The car was a kind of cramped torture where someone always had to be awake to drive, and stopping for anything, a Coke, the bathroom, or dinner, meant just that much more time on the road.

As I was packing up the Christmas presents two days before we were to leave, Hedy discovered there were no packages for Mom. I hadn't been able to force myself to buy her anything. Nothing made sense. She couldn't read or write anymore. All her meals were provided. She had lots of clothes. She only had a room with a bed, a chair, and a dresser. The Methodist Home provided everything she needed. Whenever we even bought her fancy hand lotion it quickly disappeared and was replaced by something prescribed by her doctor. Also, the last time we brought her a present it was a disaster. She wouldn't take it at first, then became upset and angry when one of the kids started unwrapping it for her. In the end, she kept the ribbon the package had been tied in and gave us back the gift.

In Hedy's clearly chiseled world of right and good, going to visit Grandma at Christmas without taking her a gift was out of the question. It made no sense to try to explain to Hedy that Grandma, my REAL mom

who loved presents, was gone. The only real Grandma
Hedy had known was the one we were going to visit.
"What should we get her," I asked.

Getting wasn't good enough. Hedy decided we
should make her a doll, a soft doll, because Grandma
loved dolls.

Hedy took charge. Together we created a rag
doll of sorts with an embroidered face and buttons
for eyes. We made it from unbleached muslin. It
looked a lot like a large, soft, unbaked gingerbread
cookie. Hedy added short, knotted gray yarn for hair
and we found a dress in our stash of doll clothes. I
embroidered Mom's name on the back of the doll so
the staff would know it was hers.

We decided not to gift wrap it given our most
recent gift-giving fiasco. We brought it unwrapped
to Mom on Christmas Day. When Hedy held it out to
her, Mom's face lit up and she took it. She kissed the
doll and cooed, rubbing it against her cheek. "I like,"
she said, "I like her."

For the next few days, she always had the doll in
her arms when we visited her. One day, however,
when Hedy and I went alone to see Mom, she didn't
have the doll with her. It was sitting on her chair
in her room.

Hedy picked the doll up and walked over to Mom
to give it to her. Without any warning, Mom took the
doll with one hand and swung at Hedy with the other.
She hit Hedy, a square sure body blow, but didn't knock
her down. Tears welled up in Hedy's eyes. She was
hurt both inside and out.

What do you say? Mom didn't mean to do it. She
really loves you. I know, Hedy, she loves you. Maybe
she thought you were trying to take the doll. She loves
the doll. She loves you, Hedy, I know she loves you.

161

POSTSCRIPT

How do you end a book like this? The obvious answer seems to be at my mother's death. Because that will be the "end" for us in our struggle with and for her.

But, I have chosen to end with my mother's life still intact. I have made a conscious decision to not "wrap the package" with a neat ribbon, a tight ending. Because the "end" of Alzheimer's is as ragged and illusive as the various "stages."

For now it feels like my mother will live forever, and we will be wrestling forever with her disease, her inch-by-inch destruction. It feels never ending. It feels without hope.

Although she does not remember any of us or our visits, we continue to go to Michigan to see her. My children are able to brace themselves for the visits. They sit with her, hold her hand, push her in her wheelchair down the halls of the Methodist Home, and try to talk to her. My two nephews, who live in Chelsea and feel her presence daily, no longer like or want to visit with her. My sister does the best she can for Mom, but limits her time with her because it is just too hard to see her mother make animal-like noises, swipe at you with the back of her hand, and scream: "No, no, no."

One day, during our last trip to Michigan, nothing anyone said or did seemed to calm Mom. She was agitated and verbal, alternately screaming at me and growling. My sister had recently described this new behavior to me adding that she felt it made visiting Mom incredibly difficult. I had patiently listened to Lolly's description and reaction and told her I knew it must be hard but she needed to remember Mom didn't mean anything by what she said or did anymore.

Fortunately, my sister had opted to stay at home that day while I went to visit, and I wasn't forced to eat my words. You can rationalize that your mother is sick and doesn't mean what she says or does, but when she does it to you, it is hard to accept. I left in tears.

During the Ninth Annual Joseph and Kathleen Bryan Alzheimer's Disease Research Center Conference one presenter flashed a graph on the screen and with his pointer showed us how, if you extend the graph of life expectancy, you see the statistical chance of getting Alzheimer's move closer and closer to one hundred percent. In brief, his research surmises that there is not really a question of whether you will get Alzheimer's, but rather the increasing statistical probability of WHEN you will get Alzheimer's. In his view, if we live long enough, we will all, in the end of our lives, live without a past or a future. We will live without memory.

It is a sobering thought.

ABOUT THE AUTHOR

Carrie Knowles is an award-winning freelance writer. Her essays, articles, short stories, and poems have appeared in numerous magazines and newspapers.

Knowles won an American Heart Association award for a three-part magazine series on cholesterol. And, in 1994 she received a North Carolina Arts Council Literary Nonfiction Writer's Grant to write this book.

She lives in Raleigh, North Carolina, with her husband and their three children.

INDEX